Fast Facts About **NEUROCRITICAL CARE**: A Quick Reference for the Advanced Practice Provider (*McLaughlin*)

Fast Facts for the **NEW NURSE PRACTITIONER**: What You Really Need to Know, Second Edition (*Aktan*)

Fast Facts for **NURSE PRACTITIONERS:** Practice Essentials for Clinical Subspecialties (*Aktan*)

Fast Facts for the **NURSE PRECEPTOR**: Keys to Providing a Successful Preceptorship (*Ciocco*)

Fast Facts for the **NURSE PSYCHOTHERAPIST**: The Process of Becoming (*Jones, Tusaie*)

Fast Facts About **NURSING AND THE LAW**: Law for Nurses (*Grant, Ballard*)

Fast Facts About the **NURSING PROFESSION**: Historical Perspectives (*Hunt*)

Fast Facts for the **OPERATING ROOM NURSE**: An Orientation and Care Guide, Second Edition (*Criscitelli*)

Fast Facts for the **PEDIATRIC NURSE**: An Orientation Guide (*Rupert, Young*)

Fast Facts Handbook for **PEDIATRIC PRIMARY CARE:** A Guide for Nurse Practitioners and Physician Assistants (*Ruggiero, Ruggiero*)

Fast Facts About **PRESSURE ULCER CARE FOR NURSES**: How to Prevent, Detect, and Resolve Them (*Dziedzic*)

Fast Facts About **PTSD**: A Guide for Nurses and Other Health Care Professionals (*Adams*)

Fast Facts for the **RADIOLOGY NURSE**: An Orientation and Nursing Care Guide, Second Edition (*Grossman*)

Fast Facts About **RELIGION FOR NURSES**: Implications for Patient Care (*Taylor*)

Fast Facts for the **SCHOOL NURSE**: What You Need to Know, Third Edition (*Loschiavo*)

Fast Facts About **SEXUALLY TRANSMITTED INFECTIONS**: A Nurse's Guide to Expert Patient Care (*Scannell*)

Fast Facts for **STROKE CARE NURSING**: An Expert Care Guide, Second Edition (*Morrison*)

Fast Facts for the **STUDENT NURSE**: Nursing Student Success (*Stabler-Haas*)

Fast Facts About **SUBSTANCE USE DISORDERS**: What Every Nurse, APRN, and PA Needs to Know (*Marshall, Spencer*)

Fast Facts for the **TRAVEL NURSE**: Travel Nursing (*Landrum*)

Fast Facts for the **TRIAGE NURSE**: An Orientation and Care Guide, Second Edition (*Visser, Montejano*)

Fast Facts for the **WOUND CARE NURSE**: Practical Wound Management (*Kifer*)

Fast Facts for **WRITING THE DNP PROJECT**: Effective Structure, Content, and Presentation (*Christenbery*)

Forthcoming FAST FACTS Books

Fast Facts for the **ADULT-GERONTOLOGY ACUTE CARE NURSE PRACTITIONER** (*Carpenter*)

Fast Facts About **COMPETENCY-BASED EDUCATION IN NURSING**: How to Teach Competency Mastery (*Wittmann-Price, Gittings*)

Fast Facts for **CREATING A SUCCESSFUL TELEHEALTH SERVICE**: A How-to Guide for Nurse Practitioners (*Heidesch*)

Fast Facts About **DIVERSITY, EQUITY, AND INCLUSION** (*Davis*)

Fast Facts for the **ER NURSE**: Guide to a Successful Emergency Department Orientation, Fourth Edition (*Buettner*)

Fast Facts for the **L&D NURSE**: Labor & Delivery Orientation, Third Edition (*Groll*)

Fast Facts About **LGBTQ CARE FOR NURSES** (*Traister*)

Fast Facts for the **NEONATAL NURSE**: Care Essentials for Normal and High-Risk Neonates, Second Edition (*Davidson*)

Fast Facts for the **NURSE PRECEPTOR**: Keys to Providing a Successful Preceptorship, Second Edition (*Ciocco*)

Fast Facts for **PATIENT SAFETY IN NURSING** (*Hunt*)

Visit www.springerpub.com to order.

FAST FACTS for
**WRITING THE
DNP PROJECT**

Thomas Christenbery, PhD, RN, CNE, is professor of nursing and director of program evaluation at Vanderbilt University School of Nursing. Since 2004, he has focused on teaching, research, and scholarship endeavors related to evidence-based practice. He is the author of *Evidence-Based Practice in Nursing: Foundations, Skills, and Roles* (Springer Publishing Company). Dr. Christenbery is published widely in journals such as *Nurse Educator* and *Journal of Nursing Administration*. Dr. Christenbery's courses actively engage students in critical thinking and clinical reasoning so that they may expand their roles as expert nurse clinicians who have a broad impact on healthcare. Dr. Christenbery has been actively involved in teaching and advising DNP students since 2008.

FAST FACTS for
WRITING THE DNP PROJECT

Effective Structure, Content, and Presentation

Thomas Christenbery, PhD, RN, CNE

SPRINGER PUBLISHING COMPANY

Springer Publishing Company, LLC
11 West 42nd Street, New York, NY 10036
www.springerpub.com
connect.springerpub.com/

Acquisitions Editor: Joseph Morita
Compositor: Amnet Systems

ISBN: 978-0-8261-5202-2
ebook ISBN: 978-0-8261-5203-9
DOI: 10.1891/9780826152039

20 21 22 23 / 5 4 3 2 1

The author and the publisher of this Work have made every effort to use sources believed to be reliable to provide information that is accurate and compatible with the standards generally accepted at the time of publication. The author and publisher shall not be liable for any special, consequential, or exemplary damages resulting, in whole or in part, from the readers' use of, or reliance on, the information contained in this book. The publisher has no responsibility for the persistence or accuracy of URLs for external or third-party Internet websites referred to in this publication and does not guarantee that any content on such websites is, or will remain, accurate or appropriate.

Library of Congress Cataloging-in-Publication Data

Names: Christenbery, Thomas Lee, author.
Title: Fast facts for writing the DNP project : effective structure,
   content, and presentation / Thomas Christenbery.
Other titles: Fast facts (Springer Publishing Company)
Description: New York, NY : Springer Publishing Company, LLC, [2021] |
   Series: Fast facts | Includes bibliographical references and index.
Identifiers: LCCN 2020019767 (print) | LCCN 2020019768 (ebook) | ISBN
   9780826152022 (paperback) | ISBN 9780826152039 (ebook)
Subjects: MESH: Advanced Practice Nursing—education | Education, Nursing,
   Graduate | Medical Writing | Nurse Practitioners—education | Nursing
   Research—methods | United States
Classification: LCC RT76 (print) | LCC RT76 (ebook) | NLM WY 18.5 | DDC
   610.73071—dc23
LC record available at https://lccn.loc.gov/2020019767
LC ebook record available at https://lccn.loc.gov/2020019768

Thomas Christenbery: www.orcid.org/

Contents

Contents

Preface

Faculty in schools of nursing often provide Doctor of Nursing Practice (DNP) students an outline to organize a DNP project paper. Outlines provide students an overall view of a DNP project paper and the sections to be completed. In addition, faculty typically include a rubric to help students gauge what level of work is expected to receive a passing grade on a DNP project paper. Outlines and rubrics offer needed foundational direction for writing a DNP project paper; however, outlines and rubrics fall short of providing academic guidance on how to write a robust and scholarly DNP project paper. The purpose of this Fast Facts book is to provide DNP students with resources to develop critical insights and rationale that will support them in writing an impactful DNP project paper. The book enables students to master the "why" and "how" of what to include in each section of a DNP project paper. This book guides students to effectively communicate, in writing, complex issues and solutions surrounding their DNP project topics. This book supports students' cognitive processes used to comprehend and communicate *structure*, *content*, and *presentation* for their project papers, which cannot be easily fostered by an outline or rubric. Students will be enabled to write about their project topics in a way that is logical, understandable, and relatable to other healthcare practitioners and scholars. Students will receive guidance to support critical thinking and writing skills, scholarly reflection, and sound rationale for developing each section of a project paper. This book fulfills a need for faculty who seek a comprehensive resource for students to use to develop their DNP project papers from conceptualization through dissemination of a final product.

The *Introduction, Methodology, Results, and Discussion (IMRaD)* model is used in this book to describe an overarching structure for a DNP project paper. Rationale for using the IMRaD model as a conventional structure for academic writing in the health sciences is explained. The book demonstrates how to organize an evidence-based practice (EBP) question or quality improvement project within the IMRaD model. Types of EBP questions (i.e., intervention, prognosis/prediction, diagnosis/diagnostic test, etiology, meaning) are reviewed, and how to adapt EBP projects to the IMRaD model is demonstrated. Standards for Quality Improvement Reporting Excellence (SQUIRE 2.0) are presented, and adaptation for use with the IMRaD model is included. Each IMRaD section is accompanied by specific areas of content faculty will expect to be covered in each section of a DNP project paper. In addition, each IMRaD section provides topics of discussion that students will want to have with faculty to provide a broader context and meaning for the DNP project paper.

Thomas Christenbery

Acknowledgments

I would like to thank Larry E. Lancaster, who thoughtfully listened to my ideas about this book and provided an authentic and candid critique.

1

Quality and Impact of a DNP Project Paper

After reading this chapter, learners should be able to:

1. Recognize indicators of quality in a Doctor of Nursing Practice (DNP) project paper
2. Describe how quality DNP project papers impact healthcare
3. Determine appropriate use of evidence-based practice (EBP), research, and quality improvement (QI) in a DNP project paper

PURPOSE AND VALUE OF THE DNP PROJECT PAPER

The Doctor of Nursing Practice (DNP) project embodies the essence of DNP education. DNP projects are hallmarks of nursing scholarship and practice that contribute significantly to the translation of science into clinical practice. In addition, DNP projects are collaborative, integrative experiences that promote important improvements in the implementation and delivery of patient-centered and/or population-based care (American Association of Colleges of Nursing [AACN], 2006). Ultimately, a DNP project prepares students to use the highest levels of knowledge to influence healthcare outcomes through expertise in leadership, policy enactment, education practices, and patient-centered care (VanderKooi, Conrad, & Spoelstra, 2018).

For over 15 years, DNP students have engaged in culminating program projects that characterize advanced practice *quality* and *impact*. A DNP project's quality represents a standard of excellence that reflects the development and provision of safe, effective, timely, efficient, equitable, and people-centered services to advance desired health outcomes (Richardson, 2000). The impact of DNP projects is evident in reshaping healthcare in the United States (Dunbar-Jacob, Nativio, & Khall, 2013). DNP projects impel the design and evaluation of innovative healthcare models, evaluate cost-effectiveness of care, influence health policy, and promote research-based interventions to optimize patient healthcare outcomes. To document a project's quality and impact, DNP students are generally required to write a comprehensive scholarly paper that emphasizes the planning, implementation, and evaluation components of a project. Some schools allow students to submit a curated collection of published papers, but typically a scholarly paper is required for graduation.

There are several reasons students want to write a successful DNP project paper during their course of academic study. First, completion of a DNP project paper demonstrates a student's capacity to identify and explore a significant healthcare issue and through the use of best evidence provide potential resolutions to healthcare issues. Second, by writing a successful DNP project paper, students display an advanced ability to appraise and synthesize various forms of research and best evidence. Third, DNP students conduct original and substantive work with a specialized health focus, thus the project paper helps solidify a student's expertise in a clinical area. Fourth, the project paper is the first point in dissemination of a student's culminating scholarship. The value of knowledge gained from DNP projects is incalculable and it is imperative that this knowledge be shared broadly. Fifth, a well-crafted DNP project paper often serves as a major stepping stone for student advancement to roles such as professors, authors, policy makers, and research team associates. Completion of a DNP project paper highlights a student's scholarly abilities and it is common for DNP graduates to be called upon by other experts and organizations seeking professionals with noted mastery in a specialized area.

ETYMOLOGY AND ETIOLOGY OF REQUIRED WRITTEN WORK FOR A TERMINAL DEGREE

The DNP project paper is similar in style to written scholarly products in other practice disciplines (e.g., medicine, pharmacy, physical therapy). Culminating, scholarly products in practice disciplines are conceptually associated with the term *dissertation*. Dissertation comes from Latin meaning "discussion or debate." A dissertation refers to a document that is submitted to support the completion of an academic degree or professional designation at a college or university. Dissertations, similar to DNP papers, comprise various chapters, typically: *Introduction*, *Methods*, *Results*, and *Discussion*. Each chapter consists of specified content, indicated by headings that are predetermined by a school's faculty. For example, an introduction chapter often includes separate headings for content such as problem statement, background, and literature review.

CONTRASTING AND COMPARING A DNP PROJECT PAPER AND PHD DISSERTATION

In a broad sense, a DNP scholarly paper leads to a clinical practice degree, while a PhD dissertation leads to a research-focused degree. Both types of papers lead to a terminal degree in which neither the DNP nor PhD is considered to be a more advanced degree than the other. The DNP project paper and dissertation are written to provide knowledge that improves the theoretical foundations and practice of nursing (AACN, 2015). Both types of papers exemplify arduous work on the part of doctoral students and must stand up to a high level of professional scrutiny. Nevertheless, there are salient purpose and outcome differences between the two types of scholarly works.

A DNP project paper begins with a student's recognition of a clinical practice problem or need and results in an improvement process using current and best evidence-based practices (EBPs). Consequently, a DNP project paper provides evidence of student growth in nursing knowledge and practice expertise (AACN, 2015). A comprehensive project paper is based on systems thinking and focuses on change for healthcare improvement (AACN, 2015). DNP project papers generally describe projects that aim to accomplish quality improvement (QI) initiatives, practice change programs, program evaluation, or translation of evidence into practice. A DNP project paper represents the generation of knowledge through innovation of practice change, the translation of evidence into practice, and the implementation of QI processes in specific practice settings to improve health or health outcomes. New knowledge presented in a DNP scholarly paper may be transferrable to other healthcare settings but is not considered generalizable to populations due, in part, to the absence of statistical probability based on large sample sizes.

A PhD research-focused dissertation emphasizes original and independent research conducted by a student (AACN, 2001). A PhD in nursing science dissertation indicates that students have actively created scientific knowledge and are engaged in the scholarly advancement of nursing knowledge. For PhD dissertations, students generally use quantitative research that generates numerical and measurable data or qualitative research methods that provide rich descriptive information, or a combination (i.e., triangulation) of both forms of research to study the same topic. A PhD student's research focus generates knowledge through rigorous investigation and systematic methodologies, which may be broadly applicable or generalizable to populations.

A DNP paper must reflect a substantive practice change (e.g., Promoting health for Kurdish immigrant populations using internet-based social media) while the PhD paper must reflect research-based knowledge development focus (e.g., Identifying types of social stigmas throughout the lung cancer trajectory). Both papers impact nursing and serve as opportunities for DNP and PhD student collaboration for positive change in healthcare. As a synergistic process, each paper brings specific strengths and preparation forward to inform healthcare in the process of research, redesigning of systems and processes, and improving healthcare outcomes that bridge the gaps among theory, research, and practice (Murphy, Staffileno, & Carlson, 2015). The application and translation of evidence into practice is a vital and necessary skill that must be fully integrated into the healthcare environment and the nursing profession (Melnyk & Fineout-Overholt, 2019).

ALIGNING THE DNP PROJECT PAPER WITH AMERICAN ASSOCIATION OF COLLEGES OF NURSING ESSENTIALS

The DNP project paper must be aligned with the AACN (2006) essentials for doctoral education. The DNP essentials outline eight foundational curricular elements that address the cost and complexity of healthcare systems, the expanding volume of new best practices, the political and social forces that drive policy, and the evolving models of healthcare economics. To fully report the impact of a DNP project, a student's scholarly paper must encompass the following eight AACN essentials:

1. *Scientific Underpinnings of Practice.* Effective DNP scholarly papers demonstrate the integration of biophysical, psychosocial, and analytical sciences that underpin the DNP project. Sound theory and science-based concepts are required to enhance healthcare delivery and improve health outcomes. For example, Social Network Theory (Kadushen, 2012) may be used in a DNP project to guide an intervention that fosters positive work relationships in an organization and subsequently used in the project paper to explain how the student implemented the Social Network Theory as an intervention. Integrating discussion of scientific underpinnings into the scholarly paper helps students underscore their project's credibility with consumers, healthcare providers, and the scientific community.

2. *Organizational and Systems Leadership for Quality.* DNP leaders assimilate nursing science and practice to address the complex healthcare needs of society (AACN, 2006). DNP students, as organizational and/or systems leaders, must describe in their project papers the factors that promote the use of scientific innovations to their maximum extent and effectiveness (National Implementation Research Network, 2019). Ways in which DNP students describe organizational and systems leadership include development of clinical practice guidelines, evidence-based interventions, and evaluating practice outcomes.

3. *Clinical Scholarship and Analytical Methods for Evidence-Based Practice*: Students must address essential number three in the project paper to demonstrate the skills that facilitate systems and organization-wide changes. An important aspect of a scholarly project paper consists of describing how students assured accountability for quality care delivery and identified potential ethical dilemmas associated with healthcare delivery. For example, if the DNP project is an intervention to prevent patient falls in a pediatric hospital, a student will want to include a root cause analysis (i.e., process of uncovering causes of problems) of falls for pediatric patients in the project facility as part of the paper.

4. *Information Systems/Technology and Patient Care Technology for the Improvement and Transformation of Health Care*: Because technology is central to efficient, safe, and patient-centered care, DNP students must address how they used information and technology to support their project practice changes. Describing the technology used to facilitate healthcare delivery demonstrates a student's ability to foster

technological innovation, evaluate the utility of consumer information, and identify potential legal and ethical issues associated with technology and information.

5. *Health Care Policy for Advocacy in Health Care*: Within the context of the scholarly paper, students must identify problems, associated with their topics, that are impacted by current policy. Evaluating a hospice organization's policies for managing acute pain and comparing them with the U.S. Department of Health and Human Services' recommendations for pain management is an example of policy evaluation. Students must demonstrate a capacity for interpreting and analyzing current healthcare policies to advance the goals of equitable healthcare and social justice that are central to DNP project topics.

6. *Interprofessional Collaboration for Improving Patient and Population Health Outcomes*: Given the multi-professional composition of healthcare systems, effective DNP projects require interprofessional collaboration (IPC). Janotha and Tamari (2017) provide an IPC exemplar in their article about care of patients with oral squamous cell carcinoma. A description of how DNP students help lead interprofessional teams using communication, collaborative skills, and evaluation is an essential component of a project paper.

7. *Clinical Prevention and Population Health for Improving the Nation's Health*: To understand the origin of healthcare problems, wise DNP students use epidemiological, biostatistical, occupational, and environmental data to inform their project's background and methodology. In their scholarly project papers, students must address how these data impact psychosocial and cultural influences of population-based care. For example, if the DNP project is focused on "interventions to reduce sharps related injuries," students will need micro and macro occupational and environmental data to form a holistic context for the project.

8. *Advanced Nursing Practice*: Because DNP students use expert, advanced nursing knowledge in specialized areas of healthcare, the project paper must reflect a student's ability to conduct comprehensive needs assessments, mentor other nurses in the delivery of optimal care, and guide patients through complex life transitions. Advanced practice nurse expertise empowers DNP students to promote safety and quality of care, reduce healthcare disparities, and lead interprofessional teams to improve healthcare outcomes, which are key components that must be discussed in the DNP project paper.

The critical doctoral-level skills gained through use of the AACN DNP essentials influence healthcare outcomes for patients and populations and therefore must be emphasized in the DNP project paper. Throughout this book, readers will find indicators of where to highlight the eight AACN essentials in the project paper.

IDENTIFYING A PRACTICE APPLICATION PROJECT

The success of a well-crafted scholarly project paper is predicated, in part, on the topic students select for their practice projects. Initially, when thinking about a DNP project topic, students may not consider how the topic will influence the process of crafting and writing a scholarly project paper. Given the complexity of DNP projects and subsequent papers, when selecting a topic, it is worth contemplating how a topic will affect the forthcoming writing process.

There is no gold standard tool for helping DNP students select the best topic for their projects and ensuing papers. Nevertheless, it is helpful for students to remember when considering potential topics that the ultimate written product must be *relevant* and *impactful*.

Fast Facts

A relevant DNP topic is significant and indicative of having a demonstrable bearing on healthcare and/or healthcare systems.

For example, "Should electronic scooter use be allowed in state parks?" may be an interesting topic, but it has limited significance and little bearing on healthcare. However, "What are the most important safety instructions for adolescents who use electronic scooters?" has major healthcare significance and policy implications. Topic relevance establishes that a DNP project and paper have the potential to be useful. The topic should have scientific, social, and practical relevance to patients, healthcare providers, healthcare organizations, and society. Scientific relevance means the project will help close the gap between current science and practical application to patient care (Institute of Medicine, 2001). Importantly, the topic must have relevance to the student to help sustain motivation and interest. Because DNP projects tend to address local, clinical problems, the topic must be relevant to the entity where the project's problem is occurring (e.g., rural long-term care facility).

The most impactful DNP projects change practice and policy. Impactful DNP projects influence, in enduring ways, how people work and live. DNP projects are, by design, relevant to the National Academy of Sciences' (2005) recommendation to prepare clinical doctorate experts in nursing, and therefore impact how healthcare organizations and systems operate and subsequently influence society. In considering a DNP Project topic, students must give serious thought to the relationships among a project's potential success, impact, and sustainability. How the DNP project impacts a select geography (e.g., environmental concerns in Flint, Michigan), culture (e.g., healthcare and the Navajo philosophy), timeframe (e.g., highest incidence of contagious disease over past 10 years), discipline (e.g., cost-effectiveness of medical homes), and/or population group (e.g., effects of urban air pollution on people over 65) must be identified and described convincingly in the project paper.

DIFFERENTIATING RESEARCH, EVIDENCE-BASED PRACTICE, AND QUALITY IMPROVEMENT

Research, EBP, and QI are among the most frequently used terms in healthcare; yet, the terms are often misused and misunderstood (Christenbery, 2018; Melnyk & Fineout-Overholt, 2019). With the increasing interest and mandates (AACN, 2006) to incorporate these terms into daily clinical practice, it is imperative that DNP students, as role models, use each term seamlessly. Inaccurate definitions and misuse of the three terms lead to diminished credibility of a DNP project paper.

Research

Research is defined as the collection, analysis, and interpretation of data about a specific subject (Polit & Beck, 2019). The encompassing principle of research is to answer questions for the purpose of *generating new knowledge* (Christenbery, 2018). Two primary approaches to nursing research are recognized: *quantitative* and *qualitative*. Though these research approaches are dissimilar, they frequently intersect. In basic terms, *quantitative research* is the rigorous and systematic collection and analysis of numeric data. *Qualitative* research is the studied use and collection of diverse resources, including, but not limited to, case studies, personal experience, group experiences, artifacts, cultural texts, and historical narratives (Denzin & Lincoln, 2005). The incorporation of qualitative and quantitative strategies within a single study is referred to as *mixed-method research* or *triangulation* (Polit & Beck, 2019).

Evidence-Based Practice

There are many definitions of *EBP* used across healthcare disciplines (Stetler et al., 1998). EBP, from a nursing perspective, is widely defined as "a problem-solving approach to the delivery of health care that integrates best evidence from studies and patient care data with clinician expertise and patient preferences and values" (Melnyk, Fineout-Overholt, Stillwell, & Williamson, 2010). This definition acknowledges that DNP students integrate forms of high-quality data, clinical expertise, and patient values that lead to optimal patient outcomes.

Quality Improvement

The term QI refers to deliberate and defined data-driven activities that aim at immediate improvements in healthcare processes, costs, productivity, professional development, and healthcare outcomes (Batalden & Davidoff, 2007). QI requires continuous efforts to lessen process variation (e.g., antibiotic use for type of bacteria associated with COPD,) and improve the outcomes of these processes (e.g., less cost for antibiotic use for common COPD infections) for patients and healthcare organizations. QI involves multiple stakeholders in the reduction or elimination of waste and loss of time, energy, and resources (Batalden & Davidoff, 2007).

Table 1.1 is a guide to clarify salient differences between research, EBP, and QI.

ESTABLISHING EVIDENCE

The message is indisputable: DNP students must be certain that patients and populations receive care built on the best available evidence (AACN, 2006). Evidence is defined as knowledge derived from diverse and credible sources (Christenbery, 2018; Higgs & Jones, 2000; Rycroft-Malone et al., 2004). Before engaging in a project that requires sound evidence and subsequently

Table 1.1

Differences Between Research, Evidence-Based Practice, and Quality Improvement

Distinguishing Criteria	Research	Evidence-Based Practice	Quality Improvement
Purpose	• Discover, explore, predict, or prescribe phenomena. • Verify existing knowledge or create new knowledge.	• Translate research and best evidence into practice. • Encourage clinical practice based on evidence as opposed to tradition. • Optimize effectiveness of current interventions.	• Foster immediate improvement in a healthcare setting. • Compare organizational standards to national benchmarks. • Improve cost-effectiveness. • Make workflow more efficient and safer.
Impact on Practice	• Generates new knowledge. • Contributes to theory development.	• Improve outcomes through translation of evidence into practice.	• Improve patient care processes (e.g., Optimizing sepsis care) and health outcomes in local settings.
Methodologies	• Quantitative • Qualitative	• ACE Star Model of Knowledge Transformation • Advancing Research and Clinical Practice Through Close Collaboration (ARCC Model) • Clinical Scholar Model • Iowa Model of EBP • Johns Hopkins EBP Process • Promoting Action on Research Implementation in Health Services (PARIHS Framework) • Settler Model	• Plan-Do-Check-Act • Plan-Do-Study-Act • Six Sigma • Lean Six Sigma

Historical Roots	Strongly influenced by scholars who used the scientific method in the 17th century.	Originated in medical disciple in the late 20th century.	Business and industry sectors.
Population of Interest	Populations for whom the findings may be generalized (quantitative) or transferable to select groups (qualitative).	Specific unit (e.g., burn unit at a medical center) or population (adults over 65 in rural east Tennessee county with heart failure).	Limited to specific healthcare unit or organization.
Examples	Identifying effective coping skills for young adults with cystic fibrosis. Predicting risk of HIV in young inner-city Asian males.	Overcoming administrative barriers to adolescent depression screening for school nurses. Implementation of maternal sepsis screening tool.	Improving patient adherence to colonoscopy preparation at local clinic. Decreasing patient wait time for ophthalmology appointments.

EBP, evidence-based practice

writing a project paper, DNP students must be clear about what constitutes evidence and how, as practitioners, they will use evidence in making critical healthcare decisions. Related, in part, to the complexity of DNP projects, a strong and broad evidence base is required to deliver optimal patient-centered care.

Effective change in patient care can be best achieved through the use of several sources of evidence. Generally, those sources of evidence are considered to be: (1) research, (2) clinical experience, (3) patients, and (4) context (Rycroft-Malone et al., 2004).

RESEARCH

Research is a methodical and meticulous investigation into a specific issue, concern, or problem (Polit & Beck, 2019). Because research is a systematic and rigorous endeavor, it generally receives a higher level of evidence rating than other forms of evidence such as clinical practice guidelines (Christenbery, 2018; Melnyk & Fineout-Overholt, 2019). In addition, for better or worse, research evidence often attains a perceived status of having unquestionable certainty and durability. However, unless DNP students approach research findings with an understanding that all research has limitations and is questionable to some degree, their project papers may contain serious misconceptions that may negatively influence patient care outcomes (Rycroft-Malone et al., 2004). First, DNP students need to know that definitive studies are highly uncommon. Researchers live in a relative world and proof is seldom, if ever, established (Godfrey-Smith, 2003). Research used to support DNP studies should be viewed as conditional, and the accepted current research base for practice should be viewed as temporal and constantly evolving (Rycroft-Malone et al., 2004).

Fast Facts

Throughout the project and writing process, DNP students should recheck the literature for pertinent research updates about their topics.

Second, while quantitative researchers attempt to gain a high level of objectivity, research occurs in a historical and social context. Thus, research is not value-free, acontextual, or static (Iaccarino, 2001). Because research is dynamic and influenced within a historical context, stakeholders (e.g., patients, health-care providers) will have their own interpretations and philosophical views of the research findings, which may or may not correspond with interpretations of DNP students. Because multiple interpretations of research will be held by stakeholders, it is unrealistic to believe that simply providing them with core research findings will impact or change clinical practice (Rycroft-Malone et al., 2004). Research is central to EBP, yet more than research evidence is required to change healthcare practitioners' decision processes and modify patient values to improve healthcare outcomes. Past clinical experiences profoundly influence a practitioner's interpretations of research.

CLINICAL EXPERIENCE

Clinical experience enables practitioners to amass important knowledge for the improvement of patient-centered care. Knowledge gained from clinical experience is sometimes referred to *as craft knowledge* or *practical know-how* (Rycroft-Malone et al., 2004). Craft knowledge is described as intuitive or implicit. Nurses draw on their own clinical knowledge and depend on the knowledge of other healthcare providers to inform care. Clinical knowledge is an invaluable key for integrating research into contextual boundaries of practice (Rycroft-Malone et al., 2004). DNP students must be certain that nurses' clinical knowledge is understood and made explicit for the DNP project to be successfully implemented. Evaluation of nurses' clinical knowledge, pre- and post-intervention, is an invaluable part of the project paper and is essential for appropriate dissemination of a project intervention to specific clinical settings. It behooves DNP students to invest time in the clinical field helping nurses explicate and elucidate their clinical understandings and narratives. Understanding a nurse's existing knowledge is a prerequisite to implementing best evidence into practice settings. All project papers must emphasize the clinical knowledge nurses possess in a given setting so that transferability of the project's findings may be maximized.

PATIENT EVIDENCE

Patients inform DNP projects with their personal knowledge and experiences. DNP students understand that the impact of their project implementations is dependent on the various ways patients and their families understand and respond to the interventions. Clearly, absolute generalization of research findings is unachievable when considering the unique complexity of patients within a population compared to patients within a particular study (Polit & Beck, 2019). DNP students will need to assess patients' previous experiences with healthcare, physical and psychosocial knowledge about themselves, and their values about healthcare before an intervention can be successfully implemented (Rycroft-Malone et al., 2004). These assessments are germane to a DNP project and are essential information to be included in the project paper. Without adequate information patient information, other practitioners will lack the knowledge for successful transference of a project's outcomes to the select populations they care for.

CONTEXT AS EVIDENCE

Context, the circumstances that form a setting, contains multiple sources of useful evidence. Awareness of contextual sources of evidence is indispensable in the delivery of best clinical practices. Sources of contextual evidence that are generally accessible to nurses include evaluation data, internal research findings, QI data (e.g., Plan, Do, Study, Act cycle), patient and family input, institutional knowledge (e.g., organizational hierarchy), professional networks, stakeholders, and institutional policy (Rycroft-Malone et al., 2004). Recognition of contextual sources of evidence contributes to the diversity of information that enriches the delivery of care addressed in DNP projects and project papers. Stetler (2003) identifies contextual evidence as *internal evidence* that is gathered systematically from sources within specific practice environments. DNP students need to be cognizant about how contextual data is collected, analyzed, and interpreted before integrating the data into clinical decision-making opportunities for their DNP projects.

OPTIMIZING ADVISOR RELATIONSHIPS

The advisor-student relationship is the *sine qua non* for DNP program success. Advisors in DNP programs generally assume a Chair role for the DNP Project Team. Advisors help students with topic identification and refinement, provide oversight of project progress, lead the project faculty team, and evaluate the level of project and project paper success. Working with an invested advisor advances the likelihood of completing the required work in a doctoral program. Productive relationships among student, Chair, and project team members are essential for developing and completing a well-rounded and successful project. The following recommendations may help facilitate DNP student and faculty cohesiveness

Prior to beginning a DNP program, it is wise to review potential faculty who might best serve as an advisor. If a particular faculty member seems like a sensible fit, it is perfectly acceptable to request to have that faculty member assigned as an advisor. Sensible fit is identified, in part, as a faculty member with similar interests and areas of practice as the student. Similar interests can be determined by reviewing publication topics and numbers of publications. For example, if a student's interest is renal failure in pediatric patients, the student may want to select an advisor who has published in that area and in pediatric journals specifically. Students may also review the faculty member's podium and poster presentations to determine if they are focused on compatible areas of interest. It is reasonable to ask the DNP department head the number of DNP students a faculty member has served as advisor/chair, the topics covered for each project, and the average number of years it took students to complete the scholarly project while being supervised by a faculty member.

SUMMARY

Understanding the quality and impact of DNP projects helps lead to successful DNP project papers. DNP projects greatly influence healthcare and are often deserving of widespread dissemination through publication. This chapter puts forth critical preliminary ideas that help ensure DNP projects and DNP project papers are conceptualized and created in a way that will support successful completion and further dissemination to the healthcare and scientific communities.

References

American Association of Colleges of Nursing. (2001). *Nursing research*. Retrieved from https://www.aacnnursing.org/News-Information/Position-Statements-White-Papers/Nursing-Research

American Association of Colleges of Nursing. (2006). *The essentials of doctoral education for advanced nursing practice*. Retrieved from https://www.aacnnursing.org/Portals/42/Publications/DNP Essentials.pdf

American Association of Colleges of Nursing. (2015). *The Doctor of Nursing Practice: Current issues and clarifying recommendations*. Retrieved from https://www.pncb.org/sites/default/files/2017-02/AACN_DNP_Recommendations.pdf

Batalden, P. B., & Davidoff, F. (2007). What is quality improvement and how can it transform healthcare? *Quality and Safety in Health Care, 16*, 2–3. doi:10.1136/qshc.2006.022046

Christenbery, T. (2018). *Evidence-based practice in nursing: Foundations, skills, and roles*. New York, NY: Springer Publishing Company.

Denzin, N. K., & Lincoln, Y. S. (2005). *The SAGE handbook of quantitative research*. Los Angeles, CA: Sage.

Dunbar-Jacob, J., Nativio, D., & Khall, H. (2013). Impact of Doctor of Nursing Practice education in shaping healthcare systems for the future. *Journal of Nursing Education, 52*(8), 423–427. doi:10.3928/01484834-20130719-03

Godfrey-Smith, P. (2003). *An introduction to the philosophy of science: Theory and reality*. Chicago, IL: University of Chicago Press.

Higgs, J., & Jones, M. (2000). Will evidence-based practice take the reasoning out of practice? In *Clinical reasoning in the health professionals* (2nd ed., pp. 307–315). Waltham, MA: Butterworth Heinemann.

Iaccarino, M. (2001). Science and ethics. *European Molecular Biology Organization, 2*(9), 747–750. doi:10.1093/embo-reports/kve191

Institute of Medicine. (2001). *Crossing the quality chasm: A new health system for the 21st century*. Washington, DC: National Academies Press.

Janotha, B. L., & Tamari, K. (2017). Oral squamous cell carcinoma: Focusing on interprofessional collaboration. *Nurse Practitioner, 42*(4), 26–30. doi:10.1097/01.NPR.0000513340.69567.4e

Kadushen, C. (2012). *Understanding social networks: Theories concepts and findings*. New York, NY: Oxford University Press.

Melnyk, B. M., & Fineout-Overholt, E. (2019). *Evidence-based practice in nursing and healthcare: A guide to best practice*. Philadelphia, PA: Wolters Kluwer.

Melnyk, B. M., Fineout-Overholt, E., Stillwell, S. B., & Williamson, K. M. (2010). Evidence-based practice: Step by step. The seven steps of evidence-based practice: Following this progressive, sequential approach will lead to improved health care and patient outcomes. *American Journal of Nursing, 110*(1), 51–53. doi:10.1097/01.NAJ.0000366056.06605.d2

Murphy, M. P., Staffileno, B., & Carlson, E. (2015). Collaboration among DNP- and PhD-prepared nurses: Opportunity to drive positive change. *Journal of Professional Nursing, 31*, 388–394. doi:10.1016/j.profnurs.2015.03.001

National Academy of Sciences. (2005). *Advancing the nation's health needs*. Washington, DC: The National Academies Press.

National Implementation Research Network. (2019). *About NIRN*. Retrieved from https://nirn.fpg.unc.edu/national-implementation-research-network

Polit, D. F., & Beck, C. T. (2019). *Essentials of nursing research: Appraising evidence for nursing practice.* Philadelphia, PA: Wolters Kluwer Health/Lippincott Williams & Wilkins.

Richardson, W. C. (2000). *Crossing the quality chasm: A new health system for the 21st century.* Washington, DC: National Academy of Sciences.

Rycroft-Malone, J., Seers, K., Titchen, A., Harvey, G., Kitson, A., & McCormack, B. (2004). What counts as evidence in evidence-based practice? *Nursing and Health Care Management and Policy, 47*(1), 81–90. doi:10.1111/j.1365-2648.2004.03068.x

Stetler, C. B. (2003). The role of the organization in translating research into evidence-based practice. *Outcomes Management for Nursing Practice, 7*(3), 97–103.

Stetler, C. B., Brunell, M., Giuliano, K. K., Morsi, D. Prince, L., & Newell-Stokes, V. (1998). Evidence-based practice and the role of nursing leadership. *Journal of Nursing Administration, 28*(7–8), 45–53. doi:10.1097/00005110-199807000-00011

VanderKooi, M. E., Conrad, D. M., & Spoelstra, S. L. (2018). An enhanced actualized model to improve DNP project placements, rigor, and completion. *Nursing Education Perspectives, 39*(5), 299–301. doi:10.1097/01.NEP.0000000000000384

2

Structuring a DNP Project Paper

After reading this chapter, learners should be able to:

1. Describe the purposes of the Introduction, Methodology, Results, and Discussion (IMRaD) sections.
2. Incorporate evidence-based practice (EBP) and quality improvement (QI) into each IMRaD section.

INTRODUCTION

In the early 20th century, the literary style for scientific and medical papers was unstandardized. Over the course of that century, a formal structure for writing scientific papers was established (Sollaci & Pereira, 2004). By 1980, the structure identified as *Introduction, Methodology, Results, and Discussion* (IMRaD) attained preeminence in scientific, medical, and nursing disciplines as the established format for presentations and publications. In addition to providing a standardized structure, IMRaD facilitates modular reading that enables readers to peruse each section of the article, scanning for specific information that is found in pre-established areas of a paper or article (Meadows, 1985). The IMRaD format is also the literary structure used for many research-focused documents such as grants, proposals, recommendation reports, and marketing and management plans. Note: Some suggest that the *a* in *IMRaD* should stand for *and* while others suggest the *a* is best used to identify *analysis*. In this book, *a* will indicate *and*.

Analysis will be presented and discussed as a critical component of the IMRaD *Discussion* section.

Because IMRaD is a frequently used format in scientific writing (Sollaci & Pereira, 2004), and is used across healthcare disciplines, the format was readily adopted by many Doctor of Nursing Practice (DNP) programs as a structure for writing DNP project papers. The IMRaD format is especially useful for DNP students who transfer science and best evidence into clinical and systems practice. The IMRaD format provides a structure for DNP students to objectively present a synthesis of best evidence that demonstrates a genuine interest in developing deeper understandings and applications for advancing science into practice.

The following content is a brief overview of each IMRaD unit. Because DNP project papers are generally predicated on EBP and quality improvement (QI) initiatives, the IMRaD overview will be followed by discussion about organizing EBP and QI projects within the IMRaD format. Section III will provide a thorough review of content generally expected in each IMRaD unit.

Writing an Introduction

When preparing and writing an Introduction section of a DNP project paper, students should recall a quote from Euripides, "a bad beginning makes a bad ending" (Collard & Cropp, 2008). In fact, an inauspicious introduction jeopardizes each unit of the IMRaD. An introduction serves as a reader's guide for the entire project paper. Without a proper introduction, readers (e.g., faculty) are unlikely to fully engage in the remaining units of a paper.

Introduction sections, in the IMRaD format, are often quite lengthy because they provide more than a standard introduction of announcing a topic (e.g., the purpose of this paper is to discuss nutrition in school-age children). For DNP project papers, it is typical for an introduction to be 15 to 30 pages in length. Organization, clarity, and analytical capacity in the introduction, encourage readers to continue reading subsequent sections of the DNP project paper. A successful DNP project that is presented as a project paper, with a non-systematized introduction will confuse readers and possibly remain unread. Within the IMRaD format, the introduction must accomplish the following: (1) a general topic is stated to engage a reader's interest in the subject matter, (2) current, primary literature is used to provide an up-to-date understanding of the general topic and to justify why the project is important to healthcare, (3) a problem, issue, or gap, stemming from current literature is presented to demonstrate for readers that a topic has not been adequately addressed for application in a local setting, (4) statement of the paper's objective(s), and (5) a brief forecast depicting how the problem, issue, or gap will be addressed to indicate how patients or populations stand to benefit from the DNP project. This presentation sequence provides readers with a necessary and logical introductory path for understanding the intent of the project paper.

METHODOLOGY

The Introduction section tells the reader *why* the DNP project was undertaken, and the methodology explains *how* it was undertaken. The methodology section provides readers with the methods and procedures used to conduct the DNP project. Regardless of a student's project topic, the Methods section must be clear, specific, and systematically focused on the DNP project. The methodology section provides other practitioners with information to replicate a project in their local settings or asses for alternative methods for addressing similar clinical problems. For example, if a survey is conducted as part of the project, students must supply the questions asked, the number of participants interviewed, salient characteristics about the sample, and why a survey was selected over other methods for gathering data. In the methodology section, subheadings are required to present a logical flow of detailed information about participants (e.g., staff, patients, community leaders), setting, equipment, materials, procedures, and interventions. In addition to detailed information, justification for selecting all aspects of the Methods section must be included. Complications encountered while conducting the project, such as high attrition rate of participants, are included in the Methods section. While providing such detail may seem tedious, students need to remember that attention to detail in the Methods section is an excellent way to ensure that readers understand that a project is valid, reliable, and trustworthy.

Fast Facts

If the methodology section is sound, readers will likely find the project paper to be more convincing.

RESULTS

The purpose of the Results section is to display and describe the outcome information gathered in the methodology section. Similar to the methodology section, the Results section should be presented in a logical, sequenced order. For example, if a student places a survey first in the Methods section followed by a focus group description, the items should be presented respectively in the Results section. Results are presented in a straightforward manner without analysis, interpretation, or bias. The Results section helps draw readers toward upcoming conclusions provided in the Discussion section. A Results section may include percentages and averages of findings, quotes, interview summaries, description of observational data, and charts, graphs, or tables. DNP students need to provide detailed results information that has relevance to the EBP or QI initiative for the project. Frequently, the Results section is short, depending on the amount of data needed to adequately identify and describe the outcomes.

DISCUSSION

The *analysis* of data, presented in the Results section, is included as part of the Discussion section. The goal of data analysis in the DNP project is to discover useful information within the data to support clinical decision-making related to the project. Data from various sources are examined, and using logical reasoning and analytical skills, conclusions are made about the data. Typically, an analysis depicts what was learned from the data. Analysis provides a DNP student an opportunity to help readers make critical conceptual linkages. For example, what do grade-school teachers report about a school-based *civility* intervention in reducing student-to-student *aggression* at recess? Or, in an oncology clinic, did clinic appointment *adherence* improve after a *health literacy* program was initiated? In the analysis section, students should draw only those conclusions that the evidence suggests. It would be inappropriate, and possibly jeopardize patient care, to make unconfirmed inferences.

Similar to the introduction, the discussion carries a significant amount of importance beyond a short conclusion. In addition to summarizing the findings, DNP students must make substantiated cases for why the project's findings or outcomes are accurate and why the outcomes are important to patients, healthcare providers, and society. In addition, DNP students need to discuss limitations noted during the project that may have affected the outcomes. It is especially important to discuss if any limitations were anticipated and how those potential limitations were addressed. Finally, students need to address what additional projects or studies, if any, should be conducted to further address the initial clinical problem.

ORGANIZING EVIDENCE-BASED PRACTICE AND QUALITY IMPROVEMENT WITHIN IMRaD

DNP projects should focus on initiatives and interventions that promote quality of care and safety for patients and populations (White, Dudley-Brown, & Terhaar, 2016). Evidence-based practice (EBP) and QI are two primary methods DNP students use to integrate science into practice and improve health outcomes through process changes in specific settings (e.g., QI). EBP and QI projects are highly adaptable to the IMRaD format. It is important to use the IMRaD format for reporting EBP and QI because the IMRaD format: (1) organizes the EBP and QI projects in an efficient and methodical way to provide essential information for readers to evaluate outcomes for possible use in their clinical settings, (2) helps ensure that students are including all essential information within the text of project papers, (3) serves as a logical guide and design for organizing the project paper, and (4) increases the likelihood that the project paper will be more easily adaptable for professional journals that require the IMRaD format for publication (Oermann, Christenbery, & Turner, 2018; Oermann, Turner, & Carmen, 2014).

Regardless of whether a DNP project is predicated on EBP or QI, the project paper format must be planned early so that essential and required information is gathered, retained, and positioned in a logical arrangement. Organization of EBP or QI projects within the IMRaD format helps ensure that later dissemination of the project at conferences or in publications is accomplished successfully.

Fast Facts

Without logical and proper documentation of each project element, readers and reviewers may raise questions about the validity of the project for application to practice.

ORGANIZING THE DNP PROJECT PAPER USING EVIDENCE-BASED PRACTICE

DNP graduates have a critical role in the transfer of knowledge to practice (Moore & Watters, 2013). EBP is a method frequently used by DNP students to systematically implement best science and evidence for making clinical practice changes. Seven steps are commonly recognized in the EBP process: (1) Cultivate a spirit of inquiry, (2) formulate questions, (3) find the best evidence, (4) appraise the evidence, (5) implement the evidence, (6) evaluate the outcome, and (7) disseminate the evidence (Melnyk & Fineout-Overholt, 2019). Each of these steps corresponds to a specific IMRaD section. **Note:** It is important to remember that each EBP step does not complete an IMRaD section. Each section of the IMRaD will require additional standardized information, which will be discussed in Section III. The purpose of Table 2.1 is to provide students an easy conceptualization of where the steps of their EBP projects will fit within the IMRaD format (Table 2.1).

ORGANIZING THE DNP PROJECT PAPER USING QUALITY IMPROVEMENT

The Standards for Quality Improvement Reporting Excellence 2.0 (SQUIRE 2.0) guidelines are easily adaptable to the IMRaD format. SQUIRE 2.0 guidelines help ensure that QI studies are comprehensive, orderly, and usable (Oermann, 2009). SQUIRE 2.0 guidelines are especially germane to DNP student QI projects. SQUIRE 2.0 guidelines are specifically designed to describe QI system level work to improve quality and safety of patient care and help establish that observed outcomes are related to an intervention. Students who use SQUIRE 2.0 in the IMRaD format are enabled to develop project papers that provide readers with the necessary detailed descriptions of the project problem, context, intervention, and outcomes. Table 2.2 depicts SQUIRE 2.0 guidelines within the IMRaD format.

SQUIRE 2.0 guidelines are an efficient and effective method for reporting quality improvement work. The guidelines were designed to fit the IMRaD format and should follow a similar pattern for the DNP project paper. If the SQUIRE 2.0 guidelines are followed carefully, students will likely find an easier transition from project paper to professional publication, since most healthcare publications are formatted using the IMRaD format.

Table 2.1

Organizing EBP Within IMRaD

IMRaD Section	EBP Step	Discussion	Example
Introduction	Step 1: *Cultivate a spirit of inquiry.*	*Early* in the Introduction section, students need to discuss their passion, or *spirit of inquiry*, for a project topic. A spirit of inquiry refers to an enduring inquisitiveness to find the best evidence that addresses a specific problem about a topic of interest. The discussion will include a personal description of the conditions or circumstances that inspired a student's commitment to the topic of interest.	Many patients, over age 65, seen in our primary care clinic express concern about diminishing physical flexibility. I began asking patients, over 65, who did not have diminishing flexibility issues to tell me about their weekly physical activities. Several patients mentioned attending yoga classes as part of their weekly physical activities.
Introduction	Step 2: *Formulate a clinical question.*	The scholarly project and project paper are predicated on a well-crafted clinical question, which helps students to focus their efforts on addressing the key issue or problem and its key concepts. Generally, the clinical question originates from patient care encounters that generates questions about intervention, diagnosis, etiology, prevention, prognosis/prediction, quality of life/meaning, and treatments. In EBP, the question takes the PICOT format.	In patients over 65 years of age (P), does a weekly 1-hour restorative yoga session (I) compared with patients who do not receive restorative yoga sessions (C) lessen sensations of physical inflexibility (O) after one month (T)?

(continued)

Chapter **2** **Structuring a DNP Project Paper**

Table 2.1

Organizing EBP Within IMRaD (continued)

Method	Step 3: *Find the best available evidence.*	Step three is a methodical search for the most relevant evidence. Discussion in this section will include: (1) identifying key search terms, including terms in the PICOT question, (2) selecting reputable search resources, such as PubMed, CINAHL, and the Cochrane Library, and then formulating an effective search strategy using MESH terms and limitations of the findings.	Using the above PICOT question, a student would enter and combine key terms into the search data bases to locate relevant articles.
Method	Step 4: *Appraise the evidence.*	Critical appraisal is a necessary step for filtering and ranking levels of evidence.	Critical appraisal of evidence answers such questions as: • Did the study adequately address the PICOT question? • Were the study methods valid? • What were the study outcomes? • How can the study support the DNP project?
Method	Step 5: *Implement the evidence.*	Combining the best evidence with student expertise and patient values, clinical decisions or practice changes are made.	Assuming evidence indicated that supported (e.g., props) stretching can improve flexibility in the elderly, the student may implement the intervention at the clinic as a weekly group session.

Results	Step 6: *Evaluate the outcome.*	At Step 6, a student evaluates the efficacy of the implementation in direct relation to clinical care.	Step 6 will enable a student to answer if the restorative yoga should be continued as an intervention and if the intervention could be improved in any way.
Discussion	Step 7: *Dissemination of EBP results.*	The DNP project paper is one method of dissemination; however, students should also consider conference poster and professional podium presentations, publications, and presentations for general audiences.	Submission of DNP project paper.

DNP, Doctor of Nursing Practice; EBP, evidence-based practice; IMRaD, introduction, methodology, results, and discussion

Source: Christenbery, T. (2018). *Evidence-based practice in nursing: foundations, skills, and roles.* New York, NY: Springer Publishing Company

Chapter 2 Structuring a DNP Project Paper

Table 2.2

Organizing Quality Improvement in IMRaD

IMRaD Sections	Description
Introduction (Answers: Why was the project initiated?)	
Problem description	• Describes the nature and significance of a local problem addressed in the project. • Notes a disruption or dysfunction in the delivery of healthcare service that unfavorably affects patients, staff, or organizational systems and prevents care from reaching optimal potential.
Available knowledge	• Summarizes what is currently known about the identified problem. • Includes relevant research and QI studies.
Rationale	• Includes models, frameworks, concepts, and theories that help describe or explain the problem and provide sound conceptual underpinnings for potential interventions (i.e., activities or tools used to optimize performance) and help explain why the interventions are expected to be useful.
Specific aims	• States succinctly the purpose of the improvement project.
Methods (Answers: What was done?)	
Context	• Identifies salient contextual elements. • Includes the physical and sociocultural elements (e.g., education, language, technology) of a local setting.
Interventions	• Describes intervention in sufficient detail so that improvement study can be replicated in other settings. • Characterizes the project's work team (e.g., RN, LPN, MD).
Study of the interventions	• Includes description of how intervention is evaluated for effectiveness. • Presents competing explanations for observed outcomes.

IMRaD Sections	Description
Measures	• Identifies process and outcomes measures, and the rationale for selecting the specific measures needs to be stated. • Operational definitions of the measures must be identified as well as the validity and reliability properties of each measure. • Describes ongoing assessment of relevant contextual elements. • Describes methods, such as inter-rater reliability that were used to assure completeness and accuracy of the data.
Analysis	• Identifies inferences drawn from improvement project outcomes. • Identifies methods for understanding variations in the data, such as the effects of time or population attributes.
Ethical considerations	• Describes maintenance of ethical integrity including potential conflicts of interest and possible IRB approval.

Results

(Answers: What outcomes were discovered in the improvement project?)

Results	• Identifies beginning elements of the invention and evaluation, such as modifications made to the intervention and rationale for modifications. • Include details of the process measure and outcomes. • Describes contextual elements that interacted with the intervention. • Describes unintended consequences or unexpected benefits and what those may be attributed to. • Explains missing data.

Discussion

(Answers: What do the outcomes mean?)

Summary	• Identifies the primary findings and connection of the findings to specific aims of the improvement project. • Names the particular strengths of the project.
Interpretation	• Describes outcomes in terms of relevance to the intervention. • Compares the study's findings with results from other publications. • Describes the project's impact on participants and the system in which they exist. • Identifies any reasons for differences between observations and expected outcomes.

Table 2.2

Organizing Quality Improvement in IMRaD (*continued*)

IMRaD Sections	Description
Limitations	• Defines limitations related to generalizability. • Identifies factors that contribute to compromised internal validity (e.g., history, maturation). • Describes efforts used to decrease limitations.
Conclusions	• Describes the usefulness of the work and its sustainability. • Defines potential spread to other related contexts. • Identifies implications for practice and ideas for further study. Identify any potential next steps.

IMRaD, introduction, methodology, results, and discussion; QI, quality improvement
Sources: Data from Oermann, M. H. (2009). SQUIRE guidelines for reporting improvement studies in healthcare: Implications for nursing publications. *Journal of Nursing Care Quality, 24*(2), 91–95. doi:10.1097/01.NCQ.0000347445.04138.74; Ogrinc, G., Davies, L., Goodman, D., Batalden, P. B., Davidoff, F., & Stevens, D. (2016). SQUIRE 2.0 (Standards for Quality Improvement Reporting Excellence): Revised publication guidelines from a detailed consensus process. *British Medical Journal Quality and Safety, 12*, 986–992. doi:10.1136/bmjqs-2015-004411.

SUMMARY

Organized structuring of the DNP project paper is a requirement for successful completion of most DNP programs. Section II described essential construction components for DNP project papers using the IMRaD format. In addition, adaptation of EBP and QI projects to the IMRaD format were reviewed.

References

Christenbery, T. (2018). *Evidence-based practice in nursing: foundations, skills, and roles.* New York, NY: Springer Publishing Company.

Collard, C., & Cropp, M. (2008). *Euripides fragments: Aegeus–Meleager.* Cambridge, MA: Harvard University Press.

Meadows, A. J. (1985). The scientific paper as an archaeological artifact. *Journal of Information Science, 11*(1), 27–30. doi:10.1177/016555158501100104

Melnyk, B. M., & Fineout-Overholt, E. (2019). *Evidence-based practice in nursing and healthcare: A guide to best practice.* Philadelphia, PA: Wolters Kluwer.

Moore, E. R., & Watters, R. (2013). Educating DNP students about critical appraisal and knowledge translation. *International Journal of Nursing Education Scholarship, 10*(1) 237–244. doi:10.1515/ijnes-2012-0005

Oermann, M. H. (2009). SQUIRE guidelines for reporting improvement studies in healthcare: Implications for nursing publications. *Journal of Nursing Care Quality, 24*(2), 91–95. doi:10.1097/01.NCQ.0000347445.04138.74

Oermann, M. H., Christenbery, T., & Turner, K. M. (2018). Writing publishable review research quality improvement and evidence-based practice manuscripts. *Nursing Economic$, 36*(6), 268–275.

Oermann, M. H., Turner, K., & Carmen, M. (2014). Preparing quality improvement research and evidence-based practice manuscripts. *Nursing Economic$, 32*(2), 57–69.

Ogrinc, G., Davies, L., Goodman, D., Batalden, P. B., Davidoff, F., & Stevens, D. (2016). SQUIRE 2.0 (Standards for Quality Improvement Reporting Excellence): Revised publication guidelines from a detailed consensus process. *British Medical Journal Quality and Safety, 12*, 986–992. doi:10.1136/bmjqs-2015-004411

Sollaci, L. B., & Pereira, M. G. (2004). The introduction methods results and discussion (IMRAD) structure: A fifty-year survey. *Journal of the Medical Library Association, 92*(3), 364–367.

White, K. M., Dudley-Brown, S., & Terhaar, M. F. (2016). *Translation of evidence into nursing and health care*. New York, NY: Springer Publishing Company.

3

IMRaD: Introduction Content Areas for a DNP Project Paper

After reading this chapter, learners should be able to:

1. Identify key components to include in an Introduction section.
2. Clarify differences between purpose statement and problem statement.
3. Describe the importance of a Doctor of Nursing Practice (DNP) project's theoretical underpinning.
4. Construct a synthesis of literature review.

INTRODUCTION

Similar to PhD dissertations, there are no universal guidelines for determining what content, nor what order of content, to place in a Doctor of Nursing Practice (DNP) project paper. Final content selection and content sequence are predetermined by a school's program faculty. For example, program faculty may require a stand-alone literature review or require a literature review that is subsumed under a background or synthesis section. Nonetheless, the content items presented in this book are representative of content requirements for DNP project papers. Section III will outline the Introduction section of the IMRaD format (i.e., Introduction, Methodology, Results, and Discussion) and present content that is typically found in Introduction sections.

Even though faculty may identify straightforward content areas to be covered in the Introduction, this section is sometimes one of the most challenging for students to write. This perceived challenge is understandable for several reasons. First, students often experience a startling realization that the formal writing process for a culminating project must begin. Second, students are sometimes concerned about making a false start and having to begin again. Third, more than likely, the challenge comes from not knowing what to write, how much to write, and the rationale for writing each content area. To a certain degree, these concerns are addressed by a student's chosen topic, what is known about the topic, and, importantly, the clinical or systems problem a student seeks to improve. Even so, it is critical at the Introduction juncture for a student and an assigned faculty advisor to discuss these legitimate concerns.

The Introduction to the DNP project paper is characteristically composed of several sections including: (1) introductory statement, (2) problem statement, (3) PICOT question, (4) purpose statement, (5) objectives, (6) background, and (7) synthesis of the literature. To begin the project paper, DNP students generally start with an *introductory statement*.

WRITING YOUR INTRODUCTORY STATEMENT

Definition and Rationale: As a nursing scholar, you have a responsibility to describe your DNP topic within a cultural, sociological, and/or political context. Setting the context for a DNP project paper is crucial. Context outlines the form and circumstances that are relevant to your project paper's topic. The introductory statement should establish a context for readers and serve to gradually familiarize readers with the topic and identified clinical or systems problems without leaping into deeper substantive sections of the paper.

The introductory statement is a *concise* description of the topic and its related problems that you hope to improve upon. In other words, an introductory statement depicts the gap between the identified problem and your desired goal to ameliorate the problem (Kush, 2015). Readers need to understand, early in the paper, that you have identified an important clinical or systems problem and that they can expect to read realistic and state-of-the-science solutions for that problem.

A classic introductory statement is typically one page in length. The first paragraph must place the topic in the broadest possible context and serve to convince readers that the topic is interesting and important (e.g., patients from underrepresented populations often report feeling devalued and unrecognized as full participants in healthcare settings). The second paragraph describes the specific topic and should help convince readers of an important perspective (e.g., cultural humility resources for staff have not been adequately developed and applied in our healthcare clinic). The third paragraph describes exactly what was done in the project (e.g., to enhance patient feelings of respect and belongingness, a cultural humility resource kit was developed for practitioners in our clinic). Within that short space, you will address the who, what, when, where, and why about the topic. Ultimately, the introductory section should serve to entice readers to read the remainder of the paper.

Introductory Statement Example: Delivery of healthcare is often practiced with a one-size-fits-all patients approach. Because it is assumed to be efficient, Advanced Practice Registered Nurses (APRNs) may care for a patient with a specific diagnosis similar to preceding patients with similar diagnoses. However, patients present with full and multifaceted lives. Understanding and treating each patient from the perspective of their cultural heritages and lived experiences provides the potential to help patients better navigate and thrive through complex health and illness trajectories. To achieve a deeper and richer understanding of their patients, it is necessary for APRNs to understand and practice cultural humility.

WRITING YOUR PROBLEM STATEMENT

Definition and Rationale: The right problem, clearly stated and well understood, is a primary step in solving the problem (McCathren, 2017). Before a problem statement can be crafted, the problem must be well-defined (Shaffer, 2015), which is, in part, the purpose of the introductory statement. A problem statement logically follows a discussion of the significance of the problem and identifies a gap in practice. In general, an ideal problem statement will identify the negative or untoward aspects of a selected clinical or systems topic and depict why those negative aspects matter to nursing and healthcare. The problem statement needs to be clearly formulated because it will ultimately impact the healthcare organization where the project is implemented (Joyner, Rouse, & Gatthorn, 2013). Problem statements are usually summarized in one to three succinct sentences.

Sometimes, it is easy to confuse a problem statement with a purpose statement. The purpose statement will be discussed later in this section. A problem statement names the problem and identifies the problem's context and significance (Polit & Beck, 2019). Problem statements for DNP projects generally consist of the following four components:

1. *Problem identification*: What is the problem that needs to be changed in the current clinical or system environment? How was the problem identified (e.g., stakeholders, evaluation reports, chart review, staff input)?
2. *Current practice*: What is the practice context in which the problem exists (e.g., clinical, administrative, educational, informatics, policy)?
3. *Scope of the problem*: What group (e.g., clinicians, patients, families), population (e.g., Somali refugees), or organization (e.g., rural health clinic) is impacted by the problem?
4. *Gaps in knowledge*: What information about the problem is lacking and therefore impairs a solution?

Problem Statement Example: A lack or absence of cultural humility is a major risk factor for unfavorable health outcomes for underrepresented populations, such as lesbian, gay, bisexual, transgender, and queer (LGBTQ). Problems such as lack of adherence to recommended health protocols, missed healthcare appointments, and failure to schedule follow-up appointments are strongly associated with a lack of practitioner cultural humility. Because meaningful engagement with a healthcare team is essential for optimizing healthcare outcomes, underrepresented populations are at greater risk for poorer health outcomes. This project will use a practitioner-focused cultural humility resource toolkit to encourage and improve a sense of belongingness for underrepresented populations at a healthcare clinic in an urban area.

WRITING YOUR PICOT QUESTION

Definition and Rationale: DNP education is predicated on translating best research and evidence into clinical practice (AACN, 2006). It is challenging and time intensive to identify relevant research and sound evidence resources without a well-focused question. Converting information needs into a well-crafted evidence-based practice (EBP) question is an essential component of most DNP projects. Many nursing authors (Christenbery, 2018; Fineout-Overholt & Johnston,

2005; Melnyk & Fineout-Overholt, 2019) recommend a five-component template for crafting EBP questions. The five components are represented by the abbreviation PICOT: population (P), intervention or issue (I), comparison to the intervention or issue (C), outcome (O), and time (T). The PICOT question is an indispensable tool for guiding the search for best research and relevant evidence (Christenbery, 2018; Melnyk & Fineout-Overholt, 2019).

Textbooks about EBP practice provide in-depth guidance on how to develop PICOT questions (Christenbery, 2018; Dearholt & Dang, 2018; Melnyk & Fineout-Overholt, 2019). The section below is a general overview of how to create an effective PICOT question for your DNP project paper. See Table 3.1 for a PICOT template.

WRITING YOUR PURPOSE STATEMENT

Definition and Rationale: A purpose statement is a declarative summary that emphasizes the project's overall intent (Polit & Beck, 2019). A purpose statement typically begins with: "The (purpose, aim, goal, intent) of this project is to…." A purpose statement must contain the key concepts identified in the introductory statement, problem statement, and PICOT question. In addition, the purpose statement must flow logically from the problem statement. Relationships among the key concepts need to be depicted in the purpose statement. For example, "The purpose of this project is to evaluate the impact of a newly developed *pre-operative pain management education program* on *reports of postoperative pain* for patients who underwent anterior cervical discectomy and fusion."

Fast Facts

A purpose statement is generally written as one or two concisely formed sentences.

You will want to intentionally select verbs (i.e., words that indicate an act or occurrence) for the purpose statement that indicate how the problem will be solved. For example, a project whose purpose is to *standardize* a type of care compared

Table 3.1

PICOT Templates

P	I	C	O	T
Patients or Population	**Intervention or Implementation**	**Comparison or Control**	**Outcomes**	**Time**
Identify patients or population addressed in the problem statement. Include salient demographic and clinical attributes, such as age, gender, ethnicity, geographic location, and disease.	Identify the intervention, treatment, and diagnostic test that will be implemented.	Identify the usual care, control, or alternative strategy that will be compared to the intervention.	Identify expected outcomes of the intervention.	Identify the timeframe for the intervention and control.

PICOT Question Templates

Intervention

Addresses the evidence-based treatment for an illness or condition.

In _____ (P) how does _____ (I) compared to _____ (C) influence (O), _____ within _____ (T)/

to a patient whose particular ... from our sources that can address different ways of knowing ... problems. The template ... verter can also align with the PICOT question template. For example, in the PICOT ... question that is formulated from a non-therapeutic statement ... such as complementation ... or apply ... based on ... nutrition or education will obtain ... results. Similar ... to be positive ... this topic could be ... the example question ... comparison of a cultural ... intervention looking for its ... effectiveness ... than ... a ... method.

WRITING YOUR OBJECTIVES

...

Diagnosis

Addresses the act or process of identifying or determining the etiology of a disease or injury using evaluative methods.

Is _____ (I) more sensitive in diagnosing _____ (P) compared with _____ (C) for _____ (O) during _____ (T)?

Etiology

Addresses the origin or cause of a disease or condition, the contributing factors that predispose patients to a specific disease or condition.

Are _____ (P), who experience _____ (I), compared with those without _____ (C) at greater risk for _____ (O) over _____ (T)?

Prevention

Addresses how to reduce the possibility of illnesses by identifying and modifying potential risk factors and how to diagnose illnesses earlier through effective screening.

For _____ (P) will the use of _____ (I) decrease the possible risk of _____ (O) compared with _____ (C) before _____ (T)?

Prognosis or Prediction

Addresses the trajectory of an illness or condition.

Does _____ (I) Impact _____ (O) in persons with (P) _____ prior to _____ (T)?

Meaning/Quality of Life

Addresses a patient's or population's experiences and concerns about a health-related phenomenon.

How do _____ (P) identified with (I) _____ describe the experience of _____ (O) during _____ (T)?

(Comparison is generally omitted from phenomenological type questions because the patient or population will serve as its own comparison group.)

to a project whose purpose is to *transform* care suggest very different ways of solving problems. The purpose statement verbs should also align with the PICOT question template. For example, if the PICOT template used is for an intervention, then a purpose statement verb, such as *implementation* or *apply*, should be used to indicate an intervention will occur.

Purpose Statement Example: The purpose of this paper will be to describe the implementation and evaluation of a cultural humility resource toolkit for APRNs working in an urban healthcare clinic.

WRITING YOUR OBJECTIVES

Definition and Rationale: Importantly, the purpose statement provides readers with a broad overview of the general direction of the project. The objectives identify, for the reader, specific goals to be achieved in the DNP project. Objectives serve as instruction on how to achieve your project's overarching purpose. Objectives generally have a short-range perspective that serves to identify small steps needed to be taken to accomplish a project's purpose. Objectives are often created using the S.M.A.R.T. acronym (Doran, 1981), which stands for specific, measurable, achievable, relevant, and time-oriented. Objectives should make the project seem tangible by identifying how the project will be brought to fruition. DNP students sometimes categorize objectives as major and minor.

Objectives are declarative statements written in the active voice and present tense, such as, "In order to achieve the purpose, the student will (apply, construct, trial, produce, pilot) …" (Gray, Groves, & Sutherland, 2017). The DNP project objectives are formatted as separate sentences, for example, (1), (2), (3), which makes visible for the reader an orderly sequence of primary steps to complete the project. In addition, this sequence order draws attention to the objective statements as central components of a DNP project. Each objective should focus solely on one idea or theme.

Fast Facts

Objectives must be practical, doable, and measurable to help readers determine the boundaries of the project.

Objectives must not be vague statements, such as, "the student will explore the feasibility of a pilot study." Instead, objectives must be concrete and easily demonstrate how the project will be directed and eventually evaluated. In closing, it is important to remember that objectives will appear on participant surveys connected with the project as well as Institutional Review Board applications. Objectives are one component of the DNP project paper that will reappear elsewhere.

Objective Statement Example: This project is designed to accomplish the following objectives:

1. Develop a cultural humility resource toolkit for APRNs.
2. Educate APRNs in the use of the cultural humility resource toolkit in an adult healthcare clinic.
3. Conduct a retrospective chart review to determine if patients who have experienced care from staff educated in cultural humility compared to patients prior to cultural humility education:

   a. Report worrisome symptoms early.
   b. Adhere to medication regimen.
   c. Keep scheduled clinic appointments.

WRITING YOUR BACKGROUND SECTION

Definition and Rationale: The purpose of a background section to present prerequisite and/or contextual information that is vital to a better understanding of the remaining sections of your project paper. There are similarities between the introductory section and the background sections. In fact, the background section should expand upon the key ideas or themes you developed in the introductory section. The background section provides discussion context for all other sections of the project paper. Information in the background section will include the etiology of the problem, its scope, and the extent to which previous studies or projects have addressed the identified problem. The background section should identify contextual factors that may impact the project. For instance, if the project's aim is to address survivors' guilt in oncology patients, the background section should identify events occurring in oncology clinics that might impact the project. Contextual factors may include political, social, economic, philosophical, cultural, and physical features. A strong background section enables readers to determine that a DNP student has sufficient knowledge and understanding of the topic and problem, which promotes a reader's confidence in the upcoming sections of the paper.

Bear in mind that a background section is different from the upcoming synthesis review section. A primary aim of the background section is to place the problem in a broad, appropriate context, while the synthesis review is a thorough exploration and summation of relevant writings about the topic and problem.

Fast Facts

In particular, you will want to note where gaps exist in the literature, which will be addressed in the DNP project.

Background Section Selection: In the last decade, dramatic improvements in social acceptance, civil rights, and public policy for people in the United States who identify as lesbian, gay, bisexual, transgender, queer/questioning, or intersex (LGBTQI) have occurred (Hollenbach, Eckstrand, & Dreger, 2014). However, the significant health disparities that stem from persistent discrimination, oppression, and stigmatization experienced by LGBTQI individuals in both societal and healthcare settings indicate the need for further improvements to meet the needs of this population (Carabez et al., 2015; Keuroghlian, Ard, & Makadon, 2017). This is particularly salient for individuals who identify as transgender. This article presents key information about the systematic barriers LGBTQI patients face when accessing healthcare as well as how to overcome those barriers by creating safe spaces and caring for patients with cultural humility (Kuzma, Pardee, & Darling-Fisher, 2018).

THEORETICAL FRAMEWORK

DNP students generally include a theoretical framework to underpin their practice project. A theoretical framework is an orderly explanation about how phenomena (i.e., concepts) are interrelated (Polit & Beck, 2019). For example, Ajzan's (1991) Theory of Planned Behavior provides a plausible explanation of how the adoption of health behaviors may be influenced by intention, perceived control, and social pressure. A theoretical framework consists of a set of defined concepts and propositional statements that describe and/or explain phenomena in DNP projects. Propositional statements delineate and clarify relationships that occur between or among concepts. For example, a health behavior, such as cigarette smoking cessation, may be fostered by high levels of family encouragement (social support), strong beliefs in one's ability to quit smoking (perceived control), and a willingness (intention) to stop smoking. A description of the theoretical framework must be included in the DNP project paper. In addition to defining the theory's concepts, operational definitions should be provided. An operational definition describes how a specific concept will be measured. For example, obesity may be the concept, and the operational definition may be body mass index. A schematic depiction of the theoretical framework should be included in the appendix. In addition, a brief history of the theoretical framework needs to be discussed, including why it was developed and the specific population or phenomenon it was developed for originally.

Middle range theories are often ideal for describing and explaining DNP project phenomena. Middle range theories consist of a limited number of concepts and propositional statements that are more straightforward than abstract. Middle range theories, in nursing, are often specifically designed to guide clinical practice implementation.

In your DNP project paper, the following questions should be discussed:

- What is the origin of the theoretical framework?
- Are the concepts distinct and clearly defined?
- How does the theoretical framework apply to the project's population and setting?
- What phenomena does the theoretical framework seek to explain?
- What new insights or explanations does the theoretical framework offer about your project?
- What are the limitations of the theoretical framework (e.g., lack of conceptual clarity)?
- Why is the theoretical framework specifically relevant to your project?
- What implications does the theoretical framework have for practice or systems changes?

Theoretical Framework Section Example: The Theory of Cultural Humility (Foronda, 2020) was used to underpin the DNP project. The Theory of Cultural Humility served as a guide for APRNs to actively promote diversity and inclusivity in a complex clinical environment. The theory enabled APRNs to have awareness of diversity, power imbalances, and multiple layers of context that influence their cultural perspectives. According to the Theory of Cultural Humility, potential conflicts can be expected and embraced with positivity. By engaging in cultural humility, mutual benefits result between APRNs and the patients they serve. A primary concept for cultural humility is flexibility. Individuals, groups, and communities hold certain life experiences, mindsets, values, and behaviors. When cultural conflict exists, the only chance for a healthy partnership is when minimally one side is open-minded to adapting. Many times, when one is flexible, others in the environment notice this attempt and will shift to positive behaviors as well.

Fast Facts

Key concepts in the above description of the Theory of Cultural Humility include *diversity, power imbalance,* and *context*. Each of these concepts would need to be clearly defined in a DNP paper.

WRITING YOUR SYNTHESIS OF THE LITERATURE REVIEW SECTION

Definition and Rationale: Synthesis of the literature is a time-honored tradition in doctoral program scholarship (Joyner et al., 2013). The synthesis of literature for DNP projects has a key role in establishing the linkages between the translations of science into everyday clinical practice. Undoubtedly, a well-crafted synthesis of the literature is an exciting section of the DNP paper to write but also a challenging and time-consuming section to create. A persuasive synthesis of the literature requires you to conduct an extensive search of publications about your topic. After gathering the best publications, you must rigorously and systematically read, appraise, combine, and *convey to your readers* important insights and understandings about the literature.

A synthesis of the literature review is a comprehensive survey of the literature that provides a description, appraisal, and meaningful summation of what other authors have written about your selected topic (Machi & McEvoy, 2016). A synthesis of the literature describes similarities and differences among the reviewed articles and provides new and deeper interpretations about the body of literature as a whole (Bonnel & Smith, 2018). DNP students conduct their projects within the context of existing knowledge. Sound knowledge provides evidential underpinnings for your DNP project. To inform your readers of the literature search parameters, the following key elements should be discussed first in the synthesis section.

Search terms: For readers to understand the literature search plan, you will need to identify in your paper the primary search terms you used to gather literature for the synthesis. Search terms are composed of key words derived from your problem statement and PICOT question. Search terms are entered into a search engine to specify a particular topic to be searched for on the Web (e.g., Google), over a computer network (i.e., interlibrary loan), or in a database (e.g., PubMed). Search terms set the initial boundaries for the literature search. Remember that combining terms, such as *underrepresented population* and *cultural humility* with the word "or" will broaden the search to include articles about *underrepresented population* and *cultural humility*. However, combining those two terms with "and" will limit the search to only articles that pertain to *underrepresented population and cultural humility*. It is important to let readers know the Boolean search terms and modifiers (e.g., AND, NOT, OR) you used to produce the relevant search results for your project paper.

You should also list the databases used to search for articles and your rationale for using select databases. For example, "meta-analyses were sought and therefore the Cochrane Library was included as a searchable data base." Providing readers with the search terms, search engines, and databases will let them know the breadth you undertook to accomplish a thorough synthesis of the literature.

Inclusion/Exclusion Criteria: Inclusion criteria consists of the literature elements that must be present in order for an article to be included in your synthesis and exclusion criteria are literature elements that must not be present in the review. Return to the purpose and problem statements to identify and clarify scope and limitations of the search. For example, if the project serves underrepresented LGBTQ populations, you will need to clarify if that means only articles will be reviewed that include adults, adolescents, children, or all. In addition to characteristics about the sample, inclusion and exclusion criteria may include the language articles are written in, such as English and Spanish only. Date parameters for articles must be identified as part of the inclusion/exclusion criteria. For instance, "articles written between 2016 and 2020 were reviewed for this report." Scholarly work generally consists of references no older than 3 to 5 years, unless a classic work is being referenced, such as Carper's (1978) "Fundamental Patterns of Knowing in Nursing." Indicate if the literature search is composed only of peer reviewed articles. In addition, you must note journal parameters that were included in the gathering of literature, such as only nursing journals, journals from other disciplines, and/or non-health-related publications.

Results of the search: The literature search results must also be indicated in the project paper. Results of the search include number of full-text articles that were yielded and number of articles that were selected. Number of articles that were excluded should be identified, and the rationale for exclusion should be included, such as irrelevant population, intervention, and/or outcomes. The databases used should be identified, and the number of articles yielded from each database need to be identified. A flow diagram in the project paper's appendix is helpful to depict the search results. See Figure 3.1 for flow diagram.

Literature matrix: A literature matrix is an invaluable tool for summarizing and synthesizing the evidence. There are multiple formats that may be used for creating a literature matrix. Reading the works of one author will not supply adequate information about your topic and the clinical and/or systems problem. Instead you must read and critique the works of several authors. When you read the works of several authors, who are content and/or research experts in the topical area, you can compare the quality and level of evidence of scholarly works and arrive at informed insights. Keeping abreast of the articles and their findings becomes challenging when authors are numerous. Using a literature matrix allows you to see how multiple authors' ideas relate to other authors' ideas. There is no gold standard for creating a literature matrix; however, usable and helpful matrixes have common attributes, such as author/date, purpose, sample, design, results, and limitations. Typically, a literature matrix is formatted with a row for each article citation and with columns for each identified area of relevant evidence

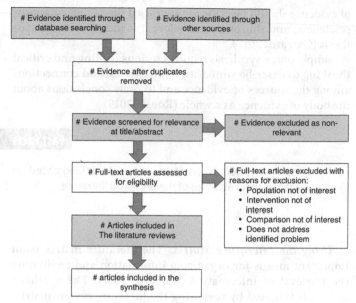

Figure 3.1 Flow diagram.

(e.g., participants, setting, design). Be certain to include the literature matrix and findings in your paper's appendices. See Exhibit 3.1 for an example of a literature matrix.

SYNTHESIS

Synthesizing the Evidence: The purpose of synthesizing is to draw new insights and conclusions about the findings in the literature. A well-done synthesis enables DNP students to identify how the appraised literature can address and inform their DNP project. A well-crafted synthesis makes logical connections among the various sources of evidence. Your synthesis section must demonstrate a critical analysis of the reviewed evidence and your ability to integrate the results. Each source

Exhibit 3.1

Literature Matrix

Article/ Author	Purpose	Design	Sample/ Setting	Methods	Instruments	Limitations	Findings	Level of Evidence

of evidence should be critically appraised for adequacy, appropriateness, and thoroughness before it is included in the synthesis (Garrard, 2017).

Simply put, a synthesis requires serious reading and critical thinking to describe similarities, differences, and connections among the sources of evidence and to draw conclusions about the body of evidence as a whole (Roush, 2019).

Fast Facts

A successful synthesis presents new ways of thinking based on interpretations and analyses of the reviewed literature.

Using the Literature Matrix: The literature matrix is an important means for organizing information and facilitating the retrieval of information (Garrard, 2017). The synthesis section is initiated by reviewing the literature review matrix, which is the summation and analysis of single articles about the project problem. To aid in the synthesis of articles, it is helpful to use an Evidence Summation form (see Table 3.2). An Evidence Summation form provides the following four key elements, which are essential to begin the synthesis:

- The number of relevant sources of evidence,
- The level and strength of each source of evidence,
- Consistency of findings among the sources of evidence, and
- Applicability of evidence findings to the DNP project.

Table 3.2

Overall Evidence Summation

PICOT Question:

Level of Evidence Strength	Number of Studies	Summary of Findings
LEVEL I Evidence from a systematic review or meta-analysis of all relevant RCTs		
LEVEL II Evidence obtained from well-designed RCTs		

PICOT Question:		
Level of Evidence Strength	**Number of Studies**	**Summary of Findings**
LEVEL III Evidence obtained from well-designed controlled trials without randomization		
LEVEL IV Evidence from well-designed casecontrol and cohort studies		
LEVEL V Evidence from systematic reviews of descriptive and qualitative studies		
LEVEL VI Evidence from descriptive or qualitative studies		
LEVEL VII Evidence from the opinion of authorities and/or reports of expert committees		

The Evidence Summation form enables students to arrange a "big picture" of the primary evidence and answer key questions that become integral in writing the synthesis. Key questions may include:

- What general statements can be made about the level and strength of the evidence? For example, are all studies non-experimental? Is there an absence of qualitative work needed to form a deeper understanding of the topic?
- How much and what type of variation in findings was noted across the evidence, especially research studies? For instance, variation in nursing care outcomes would be a primary discrepancy to identify in the project synthesis.
- Were key concepts, as identified in the PICOT question, defined consistently across reports? If not, what variations were noted in the conceptualizations? For example, *happiness* in some reports could be defined as "joy in the moment" but in other reports as "satisfaction about overall life as a whole."
- What studies or evidence best support the proposed DNP project?
- What studies or evidence provided contradictory evidence? What might those contradictions be attributed to? For

example, underdeveloped theoretical frameworks to guide project interventions can understandably lead to contradictory evidence.

■ What, if any, key theoretical frameworks were used across studies? Did the theoretical frameworks aid in defining, explaining, and/or predicting phenomena?

■ What issues or concerns germane to your DNP project were not addressed in the reviewed studies or evidence? For example, the DNP project setting may be a rural healthcare clinic, but articles pertaining only to urban healthcare clinics were found for review.

■ What key new insights and understandings did you develop as a result of synthesizing the literature?

■ What was missing from the literature that would better help to address your topic and related problem statement?

Organizing the synthesis: To complete the synthesis, it is important to identify salient *themes* (e.g., inconsistencies among study findings) or *categories* (e.g., specific attributes of participants or settings) found in the literature matrix. The literature matrix helps you to compare and contrast the themes and categories. Comparing and contrasting will help detect the relationships, or absence of relationships, among pertinent areas. For each theme or category, students should create a sentence that describes and synthesizes the identified area.

For example:
Theme: "Not only does the literature suggest that underrepresented populations feel marginalized in healthcare settings, some of the literature found that patient feelings of marginalization led to *follow-up appointment nonadherence*."
Category: "Much of the literature points out that underrepresented groups feel marginalized in healthcare settings, yet only two *experimental studies* have explored possible causes of this phenomenon."

Once key themes and categories are recognized, it is wise to outline the themes and categories with specific references. With each theme or category, you must summarize the key points to support the discussion. At the end of the synthesis section, you will need to write a concluding overview about the current knowledge of the identified project problem. Within the concluding remarks, you should address any gaps in the overall body of literature. You will want to identify any areas for future DNP projects and provide suggestions for areas of collaborative research. It is especially important for you to identify gaps between the current state of evidence and a desired state of evidence surrounding the project. Strengths and limitations should also be discussed in the conclusion. For instance, a strength may be that multiple-underrepresented populations were studied, which may support generalization of the DNP project. A limitation may be that all articles were published more than 5 years ago, which suggests there is an unexplained pause in an area of study. Refer to Tables 3.3 and 3.4 for review of introduction section.

SYNTHESIS SELECTION EXAMPLE

Cultural humility, originally described as a tool to educate physicians to work with the increasing cultural, racial, and ethnic diversity in the United States, is useful for all researchers involved in human subject research. Cultural humility is a lifelong process of self-reflection and self-critique whereby the individual not only learns about another's culture, but one starts with an examination of their own beliefs and cultural identities (Tervalon & Murray-Garcia, 1998). This critical consciousness is more than just self-awareness, but requires one to step back to understand one's own assumptions, biases and values (Kumagai & Lypson, 2009). Individuals must look at one's own background and social environment and how it has shaped experience. Cultural humility cannot be collapsed into a class or education offering; rather it is viewed as an ongoing process. Tervalon and Murray-Garcia (1998) state that cultural humility is "best defined not as a discrete end point but as a commitment and active engagement in a lifelong process that individuals enter into on an ongoing basis with patients, communities, colleagues, and with themselves" (p. 118). This process recognizes the dynamic nature of culture since cultural influences change over time and vary depending on location. Throughout the day, many of us move between several cultures, often without thinking about it. For example, our home/ family culture often differs from our workplace culture,

Table 3.3

Introduction Section Checklist

Capturing the INTRODUCTION in IMRaD

The Introduction section establishes the importance and context for a DNP project. It provides background information, explains what the project is about, and makes clear a problem statement and purpose for the project.

INTRODUCTION	Completed "Yes" or "No"	If "Yes," date completed: If "No," list steps needed to complete:

Introductory Statement:

I have:

Identified the primary topic.

Explained how the DNP project makes an important contribution to health outcomes.

Described a gap in healthcare that the project will address.

Discussed the incidence (e.g., number of new cases of disease or conditions during specified time interval) and prevalence (e.g., proportion of population who have a particular disease or attribute at a specified time or over a specified time period) of the identified problem (Centers for Disease Control and Prevention, 2012). Present incidence and prevalence information from general to specific.

Described the population impacted by the identified problem. Included population variables, such as age, gender, ethnicity, and cultural characteristics (e.g., values, principles).

Referenced demographic and clinical variables from quality resources or authoritative bodies, such as the American Lung Association, Centers for Disease Control, or the National Academy of Medicine (formerly Institute of Medicine).

_____

Addressed the burden of the problem including financial, emotional, and physical burdens. For example, "the financial burden of heart failure is well-documented but the emotional burden for caring for patients with heart failure is poorly understood."

_____

Synthesized statements from recognized leaders in the topic's field about the identified problem. For example, "The Surgeons General of the Air Force, Army, Navy, and United States are united in their concerns about high levels of tobacco product use among uniformed Service members."

_____

Determined that key terms and concepts in the title and abstract are mentioned in the introductory statement. For example, if the title is "Use of Cultural Humility Resources to Promote Patient Sense of Belongingness," use terms such as "cultural humility" and "belongingness" in the introductory statement. Importantly, faculty will expect consistency of terms to be used throughout the paper. For example, a student should not use "cultural humility" in the title and change the term to "cultural competency" in the body of the paper.

_____

Included recent developments about the topic in the introductory section. For instance, "The Food and Drug Administration approved a three-drug combination, called Trikafta, for cystic fibrosis five months ahead of the agency's scheduled release date."

_____

Used references that are derived from *primary sources* (i.e., original and originated from the primary event) as opposed to *secondary sources* (i.e., an interpretation of the primary source). In fact, primary references should be used throughout the project paper.

_____

(continued)

Chapter 3 IMRaD: Introduction Content Areas for a DNP Project Paper

Table 3.3

Introduction Section Checklist (*continued*)

Capturing the INTRODUCTION in IMRaD

INTRODUCTION	Completed "Yes" or "No"	If "Yes," date completed: If "No," list steps needed to complete:
Developed a convincing statement of why this topic is important to pursue as a DNP project. Specifically, faculty will want to see projected outcomes from addressing the problem that are in alignment with the American Association of Colleges of Nursing DNP essentials (2006), as described in Section I.	____	____
Developed the introductory statement from a general topic and issue to a specific proposed solution.	____	____
Problem Statement: I have:		
Written a clear and concise problem statement.	____	____
Avoided writing a problem statement that claims sweeping generalizations, such as "All patients with heart failure are in denial about their heart health."	____	____
Avoided the use of unspecified determinants in the problem statement, such as "A *very large* portion of patients have a *huge* misunderstanding about beta-blockers."	____	____

PICOT Question:

I have:

Checked to be certain that concepts identified in the problem statement appear in the PICOT question. ___

Identified the selected PICOT template format. ___

Provided rationale for why the selected PICOT format best fits the topic of interest. For example, if a problem statement indicates an intervention will be used, you should use the intervention PICOT template instead of the PICOT etiology template. ___

Purpose Statement:

I have:

Clarified the central topic of interest. ___

Included key identifier terms that serve as indicators to the reader. For example, "The purpose of this quality improvement (i.e., type of project) project is to use multiple Plan, Do, Study, Act (PDSA) cycles (i.e., methodology) to improve reports of patient satisfaction about medication instruction." ___

Identified all key concepts for the project. ___

Used words that reflect higher order cognitive domains to delineate the intent of the study. For example, "The purpose of the study is to (evaluate, apply, determine)." See Bloom's (Anderson & Krathwohl, 2001) taxonomy for use of higher-order cognitive domains. ___

Identified the sample and/or population. ___

Identified the project setting. Examples of setting include geographic location, clinical environment, and community. ___

(continued)

Chapter **3** IMRaD: Introduction Content Areas for a DNP Project Paper

Table 3.3

Introduction Section Checklist (continued)

Capturing the INTRODUCTION in IMRaD

INTRODUCTION	Completed "Yes" or "No"	If "Yes," date completed: If "No," list steps needed to complete:
Project Objectives: I have:		
Provided a clear delineation between the purpose statement and the objectives. The objectives should not be a reiteration of the purpose statement.	_____	_____
Developed objectives with an economy of words.	_____	_____
Avoided presenting objectives as a bundle, which is confusing. For example, "Objective (1) of this study is to determine nurse satisfaction, perception of ability, and availability of resources."	_____	_____
Committed adequate time and planning into developing the objectives. Thoughtful and well-planned objectives are critical because they underpin the methodology section. Development of the objectives must not be rushed or careless.	_____	_____

Background Section:

I have:

Identified current trends that impact the topic (Joyner et al., 2013). For example, "Rural hospitals provide nearly 57 million residents with vital healthcare services (American Hospital Association, 2020). The number of residents living in nonmetropolitan counties declined by approximately 200,000 between 2010 and 2016, which is considered the first rural population decline (Rural America in These Times, 2017)." _____

Identified and addressed new research findings and interpretations of developments that are most promising about the DNP project topic. _____

Listed other key problems about the topic that might not necessarily be addressed in the current project and rationale for not addressing these problems. _____

Made certain that all relevant historical data is shared. _____

Theoretical Framework:

I have:

Provided definitions for all concepts. _____

Matched an operational definition with each concept. _____

(continued)

Chapter **3** <u>IMRaD:</u> Introduction Content Areas for a DNP Project Paper

Table 3.3

Introduction Section Checklist (*continued*)

Capturing the INTRODUCTION in IMRaD

INTRODUCTION	Completed "Yes" or "No"	If "Yes," date completed: If "No," list steps needed to complete:
Clearly outlined propositional statements.	___	___
Included origin of the theoretical framework.	___	___
Identified concepts in the PICOT question and problem statement are identified in the theory.	___	___
Described how the theoretical framework will guide and support the clinical or systems change.	___	___
Synthesis of the Literature Review I have:		
Made sure the literature fits within the context of understanding the identified healthcare practice and/or systems problem.	___	___
Used a breadth of literature resources that include relevant work from other disciplines (e.g., social work, medicine, epidemiology, anthropology) is evident.	___	___
Identified gaps in the body of evidence. For example, is there insufficient or imprecise evidence about symptom clusters for the elderly within the first 24 hours of experiencing a myocardial infarction?	___	___

Discussed competing hypotheses that serve to explain outcomes related to the topic of interest. For example, Some view competition in healthcare markets as having no place in services intended to protect the sick while others see competition as an antidote for bloated health care organizations (Goddard, 2015)." _____

Identified areas for future projects or collaborative research inspired by the state of current literature. _____

Used quotes *sparingly*. The survey nature of the literature review and synthesis does not allow for the use of lengthy quotes. In addition, the use of quotes strung together negates the very purpose of synthesis, which is to demonstrate a student's ability to integrate findings from various forms of evidence and research. _____

Avoided use of unnecessary jargon or colloquialisms in the synthesis review. Terminology that is used by expert clinicians and scholars should be the language in which the synthesis review is written. For example, instead of writing "The patients practice *due diligence* in eating their *carbs*," write, "The patients *put forth effort* to consume diets high in *complex carbohydrates*." _____ I

DNP, Doctor of Nursing Practice; IMRaD, introduction, methodology, results, and discussion; PDSA, plan, do,E

Sources: American Association of Colleges of Nursing. (2006). *American Association of Colleges of Nursing DNP essentials*. Retrieved from https://www.aacnnursing.org /Portals/42/Publications/DNPEssentials.pdf; American Hospital Association. (2020). *Rural health*. Retrieved from https://www.aha.org/advocacy/rural-health -services; Anderson, L. W., & Krathwohl, D. R. (2001). *A taxonomy for learning teaching and assessing: A revision of Bloom's taxonomy of educational objectives*. Boston, MA: Allyn & Bacon; Centers for Disease Control and Prevention. (2012). *Principles in epidemiology in public health practice: An introduction to applied epidemiology and biostatistics*. Atlanta, GA: Centers for Disease Control and Prevention. Retrieved from https://www.cdc.gov/csels/dsepd/ss1978/lesson3/section2.html; Goddard, M. (2015). Competition in healthcare: Good, bad or ugly? *International Journal of Health Policy and Management, 4*(9), 567–569. doi:10.15171/ijhpm.2015.144; Joyners, R. L., Rouse, W. A., & Glatthorn, A. A. (2013). *Writing the winning thesis or dissertation: A step-by-step guide*. London, UK: Corwin; Rural America in These Times. (2017). *Rural America's population is shrinking for the first time ever*. Retrieved from https://inthesetimes.com/rural-america/entry/20767/rural-poverty-and-population-rural -america-at-a-glance-2017-usda-ers

Chapter **3** IMRaD: Introduction Content Areas for a DNP Project Paper

Table 3.4

Faculty Discussion Table

I have discussed the following regarding my Introduction sections with my faculty advisor	Date discussed and follow-up
• Would the Introduction section be better written as discursive or reflective? In discursive writing, a student will use reason and evidence to build a case for the DNP project. For example, a student might use a discursive style to examine the strengths and limitations of scholarly work produced about the topic of interest. A reflective style may be used if a topic is best discussed as centered on first-person experiences and supplemented with references from scholarly literature. For example, a student may have insightful experiences with the topic in a clinical setting that would help justify the need for the DNP project.	
• Determine that the project is either EBP or QI. *The project should not be a research endeavor.*	
• Would the introductory section be better written as discursive or reflective? In discursive writing a student will use reason and evidence to build a case for the DNP project. For example, a student might use a discursive style to examine the strengths and limitations of scholarly work produced about the topic of interest. A reflective style may be used if a topic is best discussed as centered on first person experiences and supplemented with references from scholarly literature. For example, a student may have insightful experiences with the topic in a clinical setting that would help justify the need for the DNP project.	

- If the problem statement passes a "relevancy test." The problem statement must be significant to patients and their health and have clear implications for improving a patient-centered problem. For example, placing healthy eating brochures at a birthing center may be a nice gesture, but it is unlikely to solve maternal dietary issues for a population. The gesture lacks impactful relevance. On the other hand, designing a peer-led support group for pregnant individuals who are overweight may have significant relevance in reducing poor maternal and child health outcomes.

- Based on the identified problem, students and faculty will need to begin discussion about the feasibility of engaging in a solution to the problem. Feasibility factors to be considered include time frame, operational, economic, technology, and legal.

- Ask faculty if there is a way to make their PICOT question more relevant to the project's topic and problem statement.

- Why a PICOT question is not a *clinical research topic.*

- If the objectives align with the overall intent of the project. While the objectives are not a repeat of the purpose statement, they should have a clear and logical linkage with the purpose statement.

- To be certain the purpose statement is in alignment with the problem statement.

- If the conceptual configuration is logical and clear between the problem statement and purpose statement. For example, if pain is described exclusively as a neurological phenomenon in the problem statement, it *should not* be described exclusively as a cultural phenomenon in the purpose statement.

- Whether the objectives will fit within the allotted timeframe for the project. DNP project completion dates are often determined by specific faculty-established timelines.

(continued)

Table 3.4

Faculty Discussion Table (continued)

I have discussed the following Introduction sections with my faculty advisor	Date discussed and follow-up
• The utility of the objectives; that is, if the objectives are met, will they be impactful in achieving desired patient outcomes?	
• The background section with faculty to be certain that all relevant concepts, theories, and terms are identified and adequately explained.	
• The background section to explain how a student's project will contribute to nursing's knowledge base. This is an excellent point for facultystudent conversation.	
• A theoretical framework should not be confused with EBP models or QI strategies. Review with faculty to be certain an appropriate theoretical framework has been identified.	
• Discuss if the theoretical framework is well-aligned with the DNP project's objectives.	
• The possibility about new ways of interpreting prior research in the reviewed literature.	
• The review, discuss with faculty if the selected literature is relevant to the identified problem. In addition, review with faculty the scope of selected literature. Students do not want a review of selected literature that is too narrow and therefore excludes relevant evidence. On the other hand, students do not want a literature review of such vast breadth that it clouds the intent of scholarly communication.	

DNP, Doctor of Nursing Practice; EBP, evidence-based practice; QI, quality improvement school culture, social group culture, or religious organization culture. The overall purpose of the process is to be aware of our own values and beliefs that come from a combination of cultures in order to increase understanding of others. One cannot understand the makeup and context of others' lives without being aware and reflective of their own background and situation (Yeager & Bauer-Wu, 2013).

SUMMARY

The Introduction section should be a compelling body of work about the intent of the DNP project. The Introduction section provides students with an opportunity to establish context for the DNP project paper. A sound and well-crafted Introduction provides a stable underpinning for the remaining sections of the DNP project paper. It enables a student to highlight the importance of the DNP project topic and to present an overview of current research and evidence about the topic.

References

Ajzan, I. (1991). The theory of planned behavior. *Organization Behavior and Human Decision Processes, 50*(2), 179–211. doi:10.1016/0749-5978(91)90020-T

American Association of Colleges of Nursing. (2006). *American Association of Colleges of Nursing DNP essentials.* Retrieved from https://www.aacnnursing.org/Portals/42/Publications/DNPEssentials.pdf

American Hospital Association. (2020). *Rural health.* Retrieved from https://www.aha.org/advocacy/rural-health-services

Anderson, L. W., & Krathwohl, D. R. (2001). *A taxonomy for learning teaching and assessing: A revision of Bloom's taxonomy of educational objectives.* Boston, MA: Allyn & Bacon.

Bonnel, B., & Smith, K. V. (2018). *Proposal writing for clinical nursing and DNP projects.* New York, NY: Springer Publishing Company.

Borrell, C., Espelt, A., Rodriquez-Sanz, M., & Navarro, V. (2007). Politics and health. *Journal of Epidemiology and Community Health, 61*(8), 658–659. doi:10.1136/jech.2006.059063

Carabez, R., Pellegrini, M., Mankovitz, A., Eliason, M., Ciano, M., & Scott, M. (2015). "Never in all my years...": Nurses education about LGBT health. *Journal of Professional Nursing, 31*, 323–329. doi:10.1016/j.profnurs.2015.01.003

Carper, B. A. (1978). Fundamental patterns of knowing in nursing. *Advances in Nursing Science, 1*(1), 13–23. doi:10.1097/00012272-197810000-00004

Centers for Disease Control and Prevention. (2012). *Principles in epidemiology in public health practice: An introduction to applied epidemiology and biostatistics*. Atlanta, GA: Centers for Disease Control and Prevention. Retrieved from https://www.cdc.gov/csels/dsepd/ss1978/lesson3/section2.html

Christenbery, T. (2108). *Evidence-based practice in nursing: Foundations, skills, and roles.* New York, NY: Springer Publishing Company.

Danso, R. (2016). Cultural competence and cultural humility: A critical reflection on key diversity concepts. *Journal of Social Work, 18*(4), 410–430. doi:10.1177/1468017316654341

Dearholt, S., & Dang, D. (2018). *Johns Hopkins nursing evidence-based practice model and guidelines.* Indianapolis, IN: Sigma Theta Tau International.

Doran, G. T. (1981). There's a S.M.A.R.T. way to write management's goals and objectives. *Management Review, 70*(11), 35–36.

Fineout-Overholt, E., & Johnston, L. (2005). Teaching EBP: Asking searchable answerable clinical questions. *World-Views on Evidence-Based Nursing, 2*(3), 157–160. doi:10.1111/j.1741-6787.2005.00032.x

Foronda, C. (2020). A theory of cultural humility. *Journal of Transcultural Nursing, 31*(1), 7–12. doi:10.1177/1043659619875184

Foronda, C., Baptiste, D., Reinhold, M. M., & Ousmane, K. (2016). Cultural humility: A concept analysis. *Journal of Transcultural Nursing, 27*(3), 210–217. doi:10.1177/1043659615592677

Garrard, J. (2017). *Health sciences literature review made easy: The matrix method.* Boston, MA: Jones & Bartlett.

Goddard, M. (2015). Competition in healthcare: Good, bad or ugly? *International Journal of Health Policy and Management, 4*(9), 567–569. doi:10.15171/ijhpm.2015.144

Gray, J. R., Groves, S. K., & Sutherland, S. (2017). *Burns and Grove's: The practice of nursing research: Appraisal synthesis, and generation of evidence.* Philadelphia, PA: Elsevier.

Hollenbach, A., Eckstrand, K., & Dreger, A. (2014). *Implementing curricular institutional climate changes to improve healthcare for individuals who are LGBTQ gender nonconforming or born DSD.* Retrieved from https://www.umassmed.edu/globalassets/diversity-and-equality-opportunity-office/documents/ceod/lgbtqa/aamc_lgbt-dsd-report-2014.pdf

Hook, J. N., Davis, D. E., Owen, J., Worthington, E. L., & Utsey, S. O. (2013). Cultural humility: Measuring openness to diverse clients. *Journal of Counseling Psychology, 60*(3), 353–366. doi:10.1037/a0032595

Isaacson, M. (2014). Clarifying concepts: Cultural humility or competency. *Journal of Professional Nursing, 30*(3), 251–258. doi:10.1016/j.profnurs.2013.09.011

Joyner, R. L., Rouse, W. A., & Glatthorn, A. A. (2013). *Writing the winning thesis or dissertation: A step-by-step guide.* London, UK: Corwin.

Keuroghlian, A. S., Ard, K. L., & Makadon, H. J. (2017). Advancing health equity for lesbian gay bisexual and transgender (LGBT) people through sexual health education and LGBT-affirming health care environments. *Sexual Health, 14*(1), 119–122. doi:10.1071/SH16145

Kumagai, A. K., & Lypson, M. L. (2009). Beyond cultural competence: critical consciousness, social justice, and multicultural education. *Academic Medicine, 84*(6), 782–787.

Kush, M. (2015). The statement problem. *Quality Progress, 48*(6), 71.

Kuzma, E. K., Pardee, M., & Darling-Fisher, C. S. (2018). Lesbian gay bisexual and transgender health: Creating safe spaces and caring for patients with cultural humility. *Journal of the American Association of Nurse Practitioners, 31*(3), 167–174. doi:10.1097/JXX.0000000000000131

Machi, L. A., & McEvoy, B. T. (2016). *The literature review: Six steps to success*. Thousand Oaks, CA: Corwin.

McCathren, M. (2017). *The problem with "A problem well stated is a problem half solved."* Retrieved from https://growthmindedcom.wordpress.com/2017/05/22/the-problem-with-a-problem-well-stated-is-a-problem-half-solved/

Melnyk, B. M., & Fineout-Overholt, E. (2019). *Evidence-based practice in nursing and healthcare: A guide to best practice*. Philadelphia, PA: Wolters Kluwer.

Polit, D. F., & Beck, C. T. (2019). *Essentials of nursing research: Appraising evidence for nursing practice*. Philadelphia, PA: Wolters Kluwer Health/Lippincott Williams & Wilkins.

Roush, K. (2019). *A nurse's step-by-step guide to writing a desertion or scholarly project*. Indianapolis, IN: Sigma Theta Tau International.

Rural America in These Times. (2017). *Rural America's population is shrinking for the first time ever*. Retrieved from https://inthesetimes.com/rural-america/entry/20767/rural-poverty-and-population-rural-america-at-a-glance-2017-usda-ers

Shaffer, D. (2015). Cooking up business analysis success. *Business Analysis Times*. Retrieved from https://www.batimes.com/articles/cooking-up-business-analysis-success.html

Shaw, S. (2016). Practicing cultural humility. *Counseling Today*. Retrieved from https://ct.counseling.org/2016/12/practicing-cultural-humility/

Tervalon, M., & Murray-Garcia, J. (1998). Cultural humility versus cultural competence: A critical distinction in defining physician training outcomes in multicultural education. *Journal for Health Care of the Poor and Underserved, 9*(2), 117–125. doi:10.1353/hpu.2010.0233

Yeager, K. A., & Bauer-Wu, S. (2013). Cultural humility: essential foundation for clinical researchers. *Applied nursing research: Applied Nursing Research, 26*(4), 251–256. doi:10.1016/j.apnr.2013.06.008

4

IMRaD: Methods Content Areas for a DNP Project Paper

After reading this chapter, learners should be able to:

1. Design a Methods section with logical structure.
2. Select an appropriate design for a Doctor of Nursing Practice (DNP) project.
3. Identify critical elements of a population and sample.
4. Outline a DNP implementation plan.
5. Describe methods of data collection.
6. Distinguish between quantitative and qualitative methods of analysis.

INTRODUCTION

The Methods section follows the Introduction section and contains several critical criteria. The purpose of a Methods section is to describe the steps you undertook to answer a PICOT question and/or address a problem statement. In the Methods section, you provide a set of directions used to conduct your Doctor of Nursing Practice (DNP) project. To begin the Methods section, start with a paragraph that describes how you will organize the section and the design you will use. For example, "In this Methods section participants, measurements, and procedures are addressed. The design for this project is based on an EBP model." This basic information provides an organized framework of what to expect and informs a reader that you have a methodical plan to present the section's material.

Similar to all sections of a DNP project paper, the Methods section of Introduction, Methodology, Results, and Discussion (IMRaD) requires scholarly writing that is direct and orderly. The Methods section provides information by which readers will ultimately judge the validity (i.e., truthfulness) of your DNP project. Therefore, each criterion of the Methods section must be presented clearly and logically (Kallet, 2004). The Methods section of a DNP project paper must describe the process and provide the rationale you used to achieve a project's outcome(s). The final draft of the Methods section is written in past tense.

The primary functions of a Methods section are to describe in detail: (1) what will be done in the project, (2) why it will be done, and (3) how it will be done (Bonnel & Smith, 2018). Method sections for DNP project papers usually consist of the following six broad categories: (1) project design, (2) setting, (3) sample, (4) implementation plan, (5) data collection, and (6) data analysis. Ultimately, the number of headings and subheadings in a Methods section will depend on the project purpose statement and input from faculty advisors. In addition, a faculty advisor will provide guidance on your school's preferred sequencing of the categories.

WRITING YOUR DESIGN SECTION

Definition and Rationale: A DNP project design is a comprehensive plan for answering a PICOT question and/or addressing a problem statement. A DNP project design includes specifications for enhancing your project's credibility and applicability. Typically, DNP projects are generally predicated on either *evidence-based practice* (EBP) or *quality improvement* (QI) type designs. In your project paper, it is important to begin the design discussion by indicating which design was selected and the rationale for selection of the design.

DNP students select EBP designs to translate best evidence into practice. *Rationale* for using EBP designs include improved: (1) quality healthcare outcomes for patients and populations, (2) contributions to nursing's knowledge development, (3) current, relevant nursing practice, and (4) confidence in nurses' decision-making skills (Beyea & Slattery, 2006).

Fast Facts

A well-planned EBP design enables DNP students to implement enhanced clinical practice and systems changes.

A variety of QI designs are available to assist students with the implementation and analysis of QI projects. The primary aim of QI is to improve a product or service (Riley et al., 2010). The Institute for Healthcare Improvement (2019) extends the QI aim or *rationale* to include (1) improve the health of populations, (2) reduce per capita cost of healthcare, and (3) provide positive patient healthcare experiences.

MODELS FOR AN EVIDENCE-BASED PRACTICE DESIGN

There are several EBP models that serve as designs for DNP projects. The EBP models have varying degrees of detail but share the following elements:

- Identify a clinical or systems problem.
- Search for the best evidence about the identified clinical or systems problem.
- Critically appraise the evidence for strength, quantity, quality, and consistency.
- Based on appraisal findings, develop a plan of action to: (1) change practice, (2) not change practice, or (3) recommend further study.
- Implement an action plan.
- Evaluate DNP project outcomes (White, Dudley-Brown, & Terhaar, 2019).

The following is a brief summation of five EBP models. There are subtle differences among the models. You do not have to know the names of all EBP models and you certainly do not need to know the refined differences among models. If your project design is EBP, you will need to select a model that best addresses your topic and PICOT question. Reading an overview of the models and discussing them with your faculty advisor will help you select the best model to fit your project.

Iowa Model: This model focuses on the sustainability of EBP, interprofessional collaboration, change implementation, and patient-centered care for clinicians at all degree levels. The model's pathway begins with a clinical "trigger" that identifies a problem and incorporates decision points with evaluation feedback loops. The Iowa Model's phases are interprofessional team formation, evidence review and appraisal, synthesis of evidence, piloting change implementation, ongoing evaluation, and dissemination of outcomes (Titler et al., 2001). An in-depth review of the Iowa model may be found at: https://uihc.

org/iowa-model-revised-evidence-based-practice-promote-excellence-health-care

Advancing Research and Clinical Practice through Close Collaboration (ARCC) Model©: The ARCC Model (Fineout-Overholt, Melnyk, & Schultz, 2005) is especially helpful for DNP students whose projects focus on building resources and training mentors. The ARCC model's breadth encompasses a range from point-of-care to the broader healthcare organization. The ARCC Model's steps include: (1) cultivating a spirit of inquiry, (2) searching for the most relevant evidence, (3) critically appraising the evidence, (4) determining if the evidence is sufficient to recommend a proposed intervention, and (5) evaluating the intervention's outcomes. An in-depth review of the ARCC model may be found at: https://sigmapubs.online library.wiley.com/doi/full/10.1111/wvn.12188

The Academic Center for Evidence-Based Practice (ACE) Star Model of Knowledge Transformation: The ACE Model (Stevens, 2004) provides DNP students a framework for comprehending the cycles and characteristics of knowledge in EBP processes. The ACE Model is particularly useful in depicting the process of translating research studies into clinical practice, which is the *sine qua non* of DNP education. The model helps students identify various types of scientific knowledge (e.g., randomized central trials, systematic reviews) but is not designed to discuss non-research evidence (e.g., clinical practice guidelines). An in-depth review of the model may be found at: http://nursing.uthscsa.edu/onrs/starmodel/institute/su08/ starmodel.html

The Johns Hopkins Evidence-Based Practice Model: The Johns Hopkins Model (Newhouse, Dearholt, Poe, Pugh, & White, 2005) is designed to support clinicians who practice in complex and fast-paced healthcare environments. The Johns Hopkins Model allows for rapid and appropriate application of current and relevant research and best clinical practices. The model's three primary steps are: (1) identify a practice question, (2) search and critique evidence, and (3) translate evidence into practice. An in-depth review of the ACE Model may be found at: https://www.hopkinsmedicine.org/evidence -based-practice/ijhn_2017_ebp.html

The Integrated-Promoting Action on Research Implementation in Health Services (i-PARIHS) Framework: The i-PARIHS Model (Harvey & Kitson, 2016) emphasizes three primary elements: (1) quality and type of evidence, (2) characteristics or context of a setting, and (3) introduction of evidence into practice. The model may be helpful for DNP students because of its strong emphasis on environmental contextual elements and the use of evidence. An in-depth review of the i-PARIHS Model may be found at: https://implementationscience.biomedcentral.com/articles/10.1186/s13012-016-0398-2

DESIGN APPROACHES TO QUALITY IMPROVEMENT

The following are tools and strategies used as designs to promote QI and patient safety for DNP projects:

Plan-Do-Study-Act (PDSA): A PDSA model is a four-step cycle for initiating and sustaining innovation. A PDSA cycle (Best & Neuhauser, 2006) assesses change through developing a plan to test a proposed innovative change (**Plan**), implementing the innovative change (**Do**), methodically observing and learning from the consequences of the change (**Study**), and determining what modifications should be made to the innovative change (**Act**). A PDSA cycle is repeated to foster continuous QI. PDSA is an uncomplicated tool and requires minimal training.

Fast Facts

PDSA is a systematic improvement effort that helps DNP students maintain methodical order over the course of their project's objectives (Agency for Healthcare Research and Quality, 2019).

Six Sigma: Six Sigma (Rudisill & Druley, 2004) provides tools to improve the capability of processes. Six Sigma has two primary goals, which are to increase performance and decrease process variation. Achieving these goals helps lead to imperfection reduction and improvement in organization profits, staff morale, and quality of products or services.

WRITING YOUR DESIGN SECTION

A primary purpose of using an EBP design is to translate research into practice to achieve optimal patient and population health outcomes. A principal purpose for selecting a QI design, to guide the DNP project, is to foster immediate improvements in a healthcare system that will ultimately impact care delivery and health outcomes. These designs can be powerful problem-solving approaches to clinical and healthcare systems concerns. As designs for a DNP project, EBP and QI are adaptable to a wide variety of patient populations and clinical settings. Selecting the right design enhances a project's integrity (Polit & Beck, 2019).

Fast Facts

EBP and QI designs serve as blueprints for DNP projects and, therefore, guide students in planning and implementing the project to achieve optimal outcomes.

Undoubtedly, a well-thought-out design is needed to create, develop, and disseminate a successful DNP project. Your selected EPB or QI design must be described in detail in the project paper. Rationale for design selection must be communicated in your project paper. A schematic depiction of the selected EPB model or QI design is helpful for enhancing a reader's understating of the model or design application to a DNP project. It is wise for students to include a schematic representation of the model or design in the appendices of their papers. In addition to writing a description of the selected design, you should also consider answering the following questions about the design:

1. What specific elements of the design help support your project?
2. Why is the design appropriate for your chosen practice or system setting?
3. Why is the design appropriate for the sample or population?
4. Are there examples, in the literature, where the design was used for similar projects?
5. How will the design support evaluation of project outcomes?

Design Statement Example: The ACE Star Model of Knowledge Transformation (Stevens, 2004) was selected as the EBP model to guide this project. The ACE Star Model was chosen, in part, because of its capacity to help identify and organize previous scholarly work about cultural humility. The model also served in the assessment and application of evidence in designing a cultural humility resource tool kit.

WRITING YOUR CONTEXT SECTION

Definition and Rationale: Context and setting, as nouns, are important and distinct elements of DNP projects. Features of settings are discussed in many DNP project papers. Conversely, contextual features are infrequently mentioned as a distinct part of a DNP project paper. Failure to fully discuss context may lead to a less informed project paper. Context comes from the Latin *contextus*, which means to weave together. Undeniably, context is critical to your DNP project paper because a project's context weaves together critical elements such as best evidence, science, literature, and data to create better methods and/or systems of patient and population care.

Context is important for interpreting a DNP project's outcomes and is essential for project replication by other nurses and healthcare providers. Because contextual features are needed to understand and synthesize findings, efforts to translate science into clinical or systems practice may fail if a discussion of contextual features is absent from your DNP project paper (Tomoaia-Cotisel et al., 2013).

Clinical interventions and/or systems changes are central to DNP projects. Because clinical interventions and systems changes are modified by context (Hawe, Shiell, Riley, & Gold, 2004), it is important that context is systematically reported in your DNP project papers. There are five recognized contextual domains (Tomoaia-Cotisel et al., 2013) that need to be methodically addressed in your DNP project paper:

1. **Practice or systems setting**: A practice setting consists of characteristics that describe the unit, department, and/or clinic that are directly related to the project's identified problem. Categories of employees and their skill mix are an integral part of a setting and must be described. Categories of employees encompass the number of nurses and other healthcare providers, support staff, various specialties that providers represent, and the part-time/full-time status of employees (Drennan et al., 2018). Clinician and staff demographics, such as gender, ethnicity, level of education, and years of service at the identified organization or unit, also need to be included in your description.

   You will want to note, in your paper, if the setting has a special designation, such as Magnet recognition. Aspects of the patient panel are important and need to be described, such as size and characteristics (e.g., 24-bed post-partum unit). Ownership of the setting needs to be identified, such as a Veteran's Administration long-term care facility. Structural capabilities and capacities, including electronic health records (EHR), QI initiatives, and program evaluation efforts, will need to be discussed as part of the setting. In conclusion, the leadership style (e.g., authoritative, participative, delegative) practiced in the setting should be included in the setting description. You will need to consider and discuss aspects of leadership philosophy used in the setting. Leadership philosophies may include transformational, transactional, visionary, and/or team-focused approaches.

2. **The Organization**: Assuming there is a larger organization than the practice setting, you will need to discuss contextual factors that impact the larger organization. Ownership, leadership styles, and structural capabilities may be subsumed under the organization. Because quality healthcare service is associated with productivity and profitability (Alexander, Weiner, & Griffith, 2006) financial factors, such as private versus public payment, should be discussed as organizational contextual factors. An organization's mission and current primary goals should be identified in your project paper. An organization's primary goals may be inadvertently in competition with your DNP project's goals. Organizational primary goals may consist of initiatives, such as implementing a new EHR system, applying for Magnet status or other notable designations, and starting large-scale QI or EBP programs. If organizational and student project goals are overlapping, or even competing, it is incumbent on students to describe how to align their project goals with organizational goals to best meet the needs of patients and healthcare systems.

3. **The External Environment**: The external environment is the atmosphere that surrounds a healthcare organization or setting and, therefore, influences the performance and quality of healthcare services (Mosadeghrad, 2014). The external environment consists of the healthcare system (e.g., Kaiser Permanente, HCA Healthcare), public policy (e.g., gun control laws), and community environment that are germane to DNP projects. You will want to include contextual community characteristics, such as availability and access to healthcare environments, degree of overall community development or decline, state of public transportation, and the general socioeconomic status of the community.

Market competitiveness among healthcare agencies, in the external environment, are economic influences worth citing in a DNP project paper. Many healthcare agencies that provide care for medically underserved populations are funded by grants and other forms of financial support; therefore, any grant funding or external funding should be included in the context discussion. The effects of local, national, and international political movements on healthcare cannot be underestimated and must be included in the contextual discussion (Borrell, Espelt, Rodriquez-Sanz, & Navarro, 2007). Payment models, such as fee for service, capitated, care management payment, or long-term care hospital prospective payment service, must also be considered as part of the external environment that directly influence patient care services.

4. **Implementation Pathway**: Multiple elements and processes impact the implementation of science into practice (Rapport et al., 2018) and must be described in the DNP paper. For example, the setting and organizational history are likely to affect your proposed intervention. A healthcare organization's history with previous transformation processes, or abilities to adapt to change, will influence the success of a DNP project and must be considered. You must also consider potential or actual operational changes that occurred over the course of your project intervention. Examples of operational changes include expanding roles of APRNs, building construction or physical structural changes, staff attrition, ongoing QI initiatives, and healthcare team communication.

5. **Motivation for Implementation**: The degree of openness that an organization's participants have for a proposed DNP project intervention is critical for the achievement of DNP project outcomes. Motivational interests for personnel and key stakeholders must be envaulted prior to your proposed intervention and documented in the project paper. The spirit of motivation among formal leaders (officially selected as a leader, such as a Chief Financial Officer) and informal leaders (a leader without an official appointment, such as a direct care nurse) must also be evaluated to help gauge support for your DNP project.

Context Statement Example: LGBTQ participants who use healthcare services at the identified clinic share a health-related common culture. For example, many LGBTQ patients face health disparities, such as suicide, substance abuse, and alcoholism, that are linked to societal stigma (Herek & Garnets, 2007).

WRITING YOUR SETTING SECTION

Definition and Rationale: Although setting is subsumed under context, it warrants a separate heading in the DNP project paper. The project paper's section on setting is a description of the local environment where a DNP project will be conducted. Discussion of setting includes the specific time, place, and circumstances in which DNP projects occur and in which data about projects are gathered. Settings may also consist of more than one site. Project settings may be physical, cultural, community, familial, or social.

Setting Statement Example: This project took place at an urban adult health clinic. The clinic is staffed by 5 adult gerontology nurse practitioners and 7 family nurse practitioners. In addition to licensed staff, the clinic employs 5 health technicians and 2 medical receptionists. Approximately 300 adult patients are seen at the clinic daily.

Project settings may be physical, cultural, community, familial, or social.

The most frequently seen patient conditions are heart failure and diabetes.

WRITING YOUR POPULATION AND SAMPLE SECTION

Definition and Rationale: DNP students need to provide relevant information about their project's *population* and *sample*. It is wise for students to distinguish between a population and a sample. In statistical terms, a population is the entire aggregate of people or cases (e.g., people, health records, DNA samples) in which a student is interested. Note: A population does not necessarily refer to people only. Members of a population share at least one common characteristic or attribute, such as disease entity, gender, or geographic location (e.g., all female patients in the United States. with heart failure). However, DNP projects generally have a narrower scope than an entire population (e.g., a more narrowly specified population might be all females with heart failure who live in Davidson County, Tennessee). A population includes all cases to whom the outcomes of a DNP project may ultimately apply.

A sample is a subset of a population (Polit & Beck, 2019) who are selected to participate in a DNP project (e.g., all female patients with heart failure at St. Mark's Hospital). A sample should possess the same characteristics or attributes as the identified population. The purpose of the sample section in the project paper is to describe why and how the particular sample was selected for a DNP project.

Population and Sample Statement Example: The *population* of interest for this project is LGBTQ adults with depression in the United States. The identified *sample* for this project is adult LGBTQ patients with depression who seek mental health service at an adult primary care clinic in Nashville, Tennessee.

WRITING YOUR SAMPLING SECTION

Definition and Rationale: Sampling is a process to identify and select the participants and/or cases for DNP projects (Gray, Groves, & Sutherland, 2017). Developing a sampling plan for a DNP project includes three primary areas in which students:

- Describe the participants who will take part in the DNP project.
- Determine how many participants will be needed and available to engage in the DNP project.
- Identify how participants will be accessed for the DNP project.

These three areas must be described in your paper's sampling plan section. In addition, you need to identify and provide rationale for the type of sampling design used to recruit participants for your DNP project. Three primary types of sampling plans for DNP projects are:

- **Convenience sampling**: By far, convenience sampling is the most frequently used sampling design in nursing. Compared to random sampling, convenience sampling is cost-effective. Because nursing phenomena are often multifaceted, many DNP projects do not easily lend themselves to random sampling or other types of sampling. Convenience sampling requires students to identify and select the most readily available participants for a DNP project. Convenience sample participants are selected because they are in the right place (e.g., breast surgery oncology clinic) at the right time (e.g., first post-breast surgery follow-up appointment) and possess the right characteristics or attributes (e.g., breast cancer survivor). Students who use convenience sampling continue to recruit available participants until a desired sample size is achieved or the pool of potential participants has been exhausted (Jager, Putnick, & Bornstein, 2017). Convenience sampling is sometimes referred to as *accidental* sampling.

- **Random sampling**: Random sampling is a selection plan that guarantees each member of a *population* has a greater than zero opportunity of being selected to participate in a DNP project. Random samples are infrequently used for DNP projects, in part, because of challenges in gaining access to larger populations, time constraints, and prohibitive cost.

- **Purposive Sampling**: A purposive sampling process is a selection method in which a DNP student purposefully recruits participants who possess characteristics based on the population of interest and who meet the objectives of the project (Black, 2010). Purposive sampling is used primarily in qualitative research and, therefore, is best used for PICOT questions that are phenomenological and rely on the EBP template that seeks to answer questions that illuminate participants' lived experiences. For example, "How do single mothers diagnosed with pulmonary hypertension see life differently from mothers with life partners?"

Once the sampling plan is decided upon, students develop a sampling frame. A sampling frame is a complete list of all participants and/or cases students can select from to be project participants (Gray et al., 2017). For example, if the population is men with heart failure, the sampling frame may consist of: (1) men over 70 years of age, (2) diagnosed with heart failure for a minimum of 6 months, and (3) live in the Southwest United States. At this juncture, students determine, precisely, the participant inclusion and exclusion criteria for their project. Establishing inclusion/exclusion for participants is similar to identifying the inclusion/exclusion criteria for a literature review. Sound rationale for inclusion and exclusion conditions should be stated for each criterium. Criteria for inclusion and exclusion for project participation may consist of:

- *Demographic variables,* such as gender identity, ethnicity, level of education, geographic location.

- *Clinical variables*, which may include presence or absence of disease (e.g., trigeminal neuralgia) or condition (e. g., smoker/non-smoker).
- Language (e.g., ability to read and write English and/or Spanish).
- Professional role (e.g., M.D., APRN, LPN).

Sampling Statement Selection: Participants were self-identified LGBTQ patients at an urban primary healthcare clinic. Participants were sampled by convenience at the identified clinic.

WRITING YOUR RECRUITMENT STATEMENT

Recruitment of a sample requires thoughtful consideration of the participants and the time and effort they will be committing to your project (Polit & Beck, 2019). Sample recruitment, as a project process, must be described clearly and in a straightforward manner. The Institutional Review Board (IRB) at the identified school and/or healthcare organization will be interested in noting the absence of unethical behavior, such as participant coercion or compromising vulnerable participants (e.g., elderly, pregnant individuals, prisoners). Discussing what worked well in the recruitment of participants and what did not work well is essential information to include in the project paper. When describing the recruitment process, you will want to discuss the following elements of recruitment:

- **Recruitment method**: Describe how participants learned about the project. There are various methods of participant solicitation and one or more methods may be used. Recruitment methods include face-to-face, poster, email, and advertisement. You should provide the exact wording that was used to recruit participants as well as the rationale for the selected recruitment methods. Importantly, students will need to describe how their recruitment tool was matched to the target audience. For instance, a recruitment flyer for adults over 65 years of age with asthma will likely have a different graphic design and wording than a recruitment flyer for middle-school participants with asthma.
- **Location of recruitment efforts**: You will need to describe where the project recruitment took place, including who approached potential participants to enroll in the DNP project. Location of where contacts were made and a

detailed script that was used for recruitment must be included. Locations of where posters were placed or where flyers were handed out and by whom need to be described. Email is a popular method of recruitment; therefore, the number of emails sent and the schedule by which they were sent out should be included in the recruitment description section. A copy of an email recruitment letter and/or flyer should be included in the appendices.

- **Contact information**: Student contact information should be included. Students should indicate how potential participants were instructed to contact them.
- **Compensation**: Participant compensation, if provided, must be described in the DNP paper. DNP students often provide a form of recompense for project participation. Students should specify the type of compensation that was offered and received and the rationale for compensation. For example, a student may provide pizza for employees who participate in a focus group during their scheduled meal break.

Determining sample size must also be considered as part of a recruitment plan. One method to determine the sample size in DNP projects is to base the sample number on previous comparable projects that used similar sampling plans. Often the sample size for DNP projects is determined by the number of available participants. For example, if a student wishes to evaluate an EBP intervention for patients with Huntington's disease (HD) and there are only 20 patients with HD at the identified clinic, it is reasonable to assume the sample will not be greater than 20 participants with HD.

Recruitment Statement Example: A flyer, describing the project, was placed in the health clinic patient waiting room. Potential participants were requested to ask their healthcare providers about specific project information. No incentives were offered for project participation.

WRITING YOUR ETHICS SECTION

Sound ethical guidelines are a requirement for all DNP projects. Readers of DNP project papers will want to see evidence that ethical guidelines are followed to protect human participants involved in the project. DNP programs generally require students to complete and submit institutional review board (IRB) applications before participants are recruited for a

DNP project. Because many DNP projects involve participants who cannot give consent (e.g., minors, patients in comas), you need to indicate who signed the IRB consent form. For example, "The project intervention was approved by the Medical Center's Review Board and consent was given by the participant's mother." A copy of the IRB application and consent letter should be placed in the appendices of the DNP project paper. If the IRB waived the requirement to obtain consent, indicate in the project paper why consent was waived. In addition to IRB documentation, you need to include discussion in your paper about the following ethical aspects:

- Describe plans for protecting privacy and confidentiality of participants.
- Discuss rationale for excluding any groups from the project (e.g., elderly, military personnel).
- Summarize any potential risks to participants and plans to minimize identified risks.
- Describe any vulnerable populations, such as:
  - Children: Include ages and assent process if needed.
  - Cognitively impaired adults: Identify the parameters of the impairment, such as coma or dementia.
  - Pregnant individuals: What portion of gestation will they be in during the project?
  - Prisoners: Benefits of the project to prisoners clearly stated.

Ethics Statement Example: The procedures for the project were approved by the IRB of the university. The project was explained to all participants. Assurance of privacy and confidentiality was emphasized with participants.

WRITING YOUR IMPLEMENTATION STATEMENT

Definition and Rationale: Planning and Implementation are two of the most important elements of the DNP project paper. Project implementation is dependent on deliberate and thoughtful planning by students. Williams (1919) noted that by failing to prepare, we prepare to fail.

Fast Facts

Inadequate preparation and planning will doom the implementation of the most well-intentioned DNP project.

In the Introduction section of the project paper, students make clear what the clinical or systems problem is and what objectives must be met to help ameliorate or eliminate the problem. In the Methods section, students describe the *planning process* for *implementation*, which requires several key steps. The implementation steps presented in this section are essential for success; however, the sequencing of the steps should be determined by the student and faculty advisors. Sequencing of the steps will be dependent, in part, on a logical timeline that students and faculty advisors decide is appropriate for project completion. Universal standardization of implementation interventions is uncommon; therefore, interventions in DNP project papers must be carefully outlined with meticulous detail. A timeline depicting the timing of the implementation and the time of project measurements (e.g., pre-intervention, post-intervention) is very helpful to include in the appendix.

Implementation process steps:

- Stakeholders: You need to identify the key stakeholders (Freeman, 1984). Stakeholders are individuals who have a steadfast interest in a DNP project's objectives and outcomes. Key stakeholders may consist of patients, physicians, APRNs, direct care nurses, clerical staff, and volunteers associated with a DNP project. In addition to identifying stakeholders, it is also important for you to recognize and rank order stakeholders' specific needs (e.g., communication, ownership, approval) in terms of the DNP project. You will want to describe the roles stakeholders had in achieving the project's goals. You need to report the stakeholders' needs and perception of project objectives. In addition, you should compare the alignment of the stakeholders' objectives with the project's objectives and discuss the degree of student/stakeholder understanding that objectives were realistic, timely, and attained.

- Project faculty advisors: Refer to Section I for an overview of a faculty advisor's role in the DNP project process. In the implementation section of the paper, you will identify the advisors and describe their roles and responsibilities. For example, "Professor Smith is a statistician and will assist in the multivariate analysis of data," or "Professor Adams is a nationally recognized author in the care of renal dialysis patients and will serve as a clinical content expert."

- Organizational commitment: The degree of commitment from leadership at the organizational and unit level is crucial and must be addressed in the project paper. You will want to describe the amount of time and resources (e.g., space, equipment, personnel) organizational- and unit-level leaders are willing to commit to the project. In addition, you need to identify how leaders will communicate their support to the organization and/or unit participants for a DNP project.

- Needs assessment: A needs assessment is required for successful planning of a DNP project. A needs assessment should demonstrate and document the needs for a specific project. Areas to include in a project paper needs assessment are financial, technical, and operational considerations. In addition to identifying project needs, you will want to describe how you assured that identified needs were met to attain project completion and success.
- Communication plan: A successful DNP project is dependent on accurate and timely communication. You will need to identify how often you communicated with key stakeholders. Project updates that advisors and stakeholders received should be documented in the project paper.
- Barriers: All DNP projects have a potential for unique barriers. Describing the barriers is critical to helping others, with similar projects, to minimize project obstacles. You need to describe the strategies and resources used to limit barriers. Resources may include human, fiscal, and technical. The success of resources in limiting barriers needs to be described in the project paper.
- Budget: A budget proposal for DNP project expenses must be created, even if the project is cost neutral. Costs incurred may include incentives for participants (e.g., lunch), staff training, computer software, software license, and travel. A cost-benefit analysis should be included if the project was too costly for an organization to support. A cost-benefit analysis estimates strengths and limitations of alternative interventions or programs to help identify other intervention options that may be more cost-effective for an organization. Most DNP programs will provide a spreadsheet with instructions on how to report the cost analysis. An itemized budget sheet should be included in a paper's appendices.
- Timeline: A project's timeline will need to be included as part of the paper. A timeline should begin with the initial planning stages and end with the project's outcome evaluation. DNP programs have temporal limitations and a timeline should realistically depict the available time it

took to complete a project. To keep a timeline organized and realistic, use Excel and prepare a Gantt chart. A Gantt chart is a graphical depiction of the project tasks to be completed and identifies resources and dependencies. In keeping with a realistic timeline, you must remember to factor in holidays, vacation, IRB submission, and conference attendance requirements.

Implementation Statement Example: A key issue for the APRN team was to develop and sustain a culture of patient-centered humility. The team identified a process for creating a cultural humility tool kit that was applicable for APRNs to use across various cultures at the clinic. The toolkit was designed with input from the clinic's LGBTQ patients and the APRN team. The purpose of the toolkit was to enhance multicultural knowledge, self-awareness, and intentional communication using culturally sensitive therapeutic skills.

WRITING YOUR DATA COLLECTION SECTION

Definition and Rationale: Systematic and accurate data collection enables DNP students to appropriately evaluate their project's outcomes (Glassman, 2017). Data collection is a means of gathering and measuring findings from relevant sources about DNP project objectives, that students set forth, to accomplish identified clinical and/or healthcare system changes. Students must describe, in detail, the type of data collected, sources of data, and the methods used to collect data.

The data collection section of a DNP paper should reflect your honesty and integrity about the data collection process so readers will understand that:

- Objectives were answered forthrightly.
- The project could be replicated and outcomes would demonstrate consistency (i.e., reliability).
- You were an honorable steward of project resources.
- Practice and/or systems changes, based on the project's recommendations, did not compromise the safety and well-being of patients and/or populations.

Quantitative and/or qualitative data are collected by students for their DNP projects. *Quantitative data* consists of numeric-based quantities that can be measured and compared. Quantitative data answers questions about "how many", "how often," and "how much," (Polit & Beck, 2019). Examples of quantitative data in healthcare include number of people who have osteoarthritis, annual incidence of near-drownings, and body mass index. The emphasis on numerical data in healthcare is profound and, therefore, it is not surprising that many DNP projects rely heavily on quantitative data to describe and explain healthcare phenomena.

Qualitative data are non-numerical and may be observable but not easily measurable (e.g., mother and infant bonding). DNP projects often use patient-centered care models in which patients are encouraged to be involved in their healthcare decision making and their personal healthcare preferences are honored. Patient-centered care outcomes (e.g., comfort, rest) are sometimes difficult to measure numerically and, therefore, require a qualitative approach to better understand the healthcare experiences of patients and families (Williams, 2015). Qualitative research allows you to better understand patient-centered lived experiences and communicate the meaningful insights gained from those experiences in the DNP project paper.

Quantitative Data Collection

There are several quantitative methods used to collect data for DNP projects. Quantitative data collection emphasizes objective measurements (e.g., body temperature, pulse rate, pertussis incidence). To support the validity and reliability of a project, features associated with quantitative methods must be presented with rigor and consistency in the DNP paper.

Quantitative data are often gathered and measured using standardized instruments such as surveys, questionnaires, and/or observational tools. A standardized instrument is considered to have well-established *psychometric properties*. An instrument's psychometric properties indicate that sufficient data have been collected on an instrument to determine how well it will measure a specific construct (e.g., pain, depression, satisfaction) of interest (Polit & Beck, 2019). There are two primary types of psychometric properties that students must describe when discussing instruments: *reliability* and *validity*. You must thoroughly describe the reliability and validity properties of each instrument used to collect data for the DNP project's outcomes. An accurate depiction of an instrument's properties of reliability and validity will demonstrate for readers that the instruments are unbiased and undistorted and capable of assessing accurate findings.

Test reliability is the degree to which a test is consistent and stable, over time, in measuring what it is projected to measure. Test validity is the degree to which a test accurately measures what it is intended to measure. Table 4.1 illustrates key features of reliability and validity that must be discussed in a DNP project paper.

Table 4.1

Quantitative Reliability and Validity Review			
Type of Reliability	**Definition**	**Example**	**Score Interpretation**
Test–retest	Reliability is established by administering the same test twice over a period of time to a group of participants.	A test for trait anxiety should remain consistent if administered at a 4-week interval because trait anxiety remains consistent over time.	The score is the correlation between outcomes at Time 1 and Time 2. • 1: perfect reliability • ≥ 0.9: excellent reliability • ≥ 0.8 < 0.9: good reliability • ≥ 0.7 < 0.8: acceptable reliability • ≥ 0.6 < 0.7: questionable reliability
Alternative form (also known as parallel form or equivalent form)	Reliability is established by administering two forms of the same test, to the same participants, with slight variation of items.	Administer two different versions of questions on an interprofessional collaboration assessment tool to the same group of nursing students.	The score is the correlation coefficient between scores on test 1 and Test 2. A score of .70 is required to demonstrate reliability.
Internal consistency (alpha, α)	The general agreement between multiple items that make-up a composite score of a survey measurement of a given construct (e.g., anxiety, dread, comfort).	The undergraduate nursing test is divided into dyspnea, fatigue, and pain. The internal consistency reliability test provides a measure that each of these particular symptom constructs is measured correctly and reliably.	Common guidelines for evaluating Cronbach's Alpha are: • .00 to .69 = Poor • .70 to .79 = Fair • .80 to .89 = Good • .90 to .99 = Excellent/Strong

Type of Validity	Definition	Example	Score interpretation
Content	The extent to which a measurement identifies all key dimensions of a construct.	A pain assessment tool may lack content validity if it only assesses pain intensity and fails to capture pain distress.	*Expert judgment* (not statistics) is used to determine whether a test has content validity. A test should have a high correlation with other tests that measure the same content domain.
Criterion	Assesses how well the extent of scores on one test agree (concurrent validity) or predict (predictive validity) on an external criterion.	If a nursing school's NCLEX-RN scores correlate highly with statewide NCLEX-RN scores, the school's scores would have high *concurrent* validity. A diabetes self-efficacy measure may *predict* how well a patient will manage diabetes self-care.	Criterion validity is generally assessed by comparison with a gold standard test.
Construct	Construct validity is used to determine how well a test (usually a questionnaire) measures what it is supposed to measure.	The construct validity of a fundamental nursing skills test is demonstrated by correlating the outcomes on the test to those found on other widely accepted measures of fundamental nursing skills.	Construct validity is verified by comparing a test to another test that measures a similar attribute (e.g., self-efficacy) to determine how highly correlated the two measures are.

For each instrument used to measure project outcomes, you will need to describe how the instrument's developers defined the major construct (e.g., pain, dyspnea, anxiety) being measured. Providing the definition will allow readers to determine if the instrument's construct definition aligns with your construct definition. Improper alignment of construct definitions will signify potential problems with instrument validity You will need to indicate if pilot studies were conducted with the instrument by its developers and who were the participants in the pilot studies. You will need to indicate if participants in the pilot studies align with participants in the DNP project on key characteristics (e.g., age, disability, gender).

How the instrument or test is scored will also need to be described. For example, "a 5-point Likert scale was used to assess the intensity of participants' attitudes toward Medicare for all. The scale ranged from *1 strongly disagree* to *5 strongly agree*." If you are adapting an instrument for your project, you need to describe what changes were made to the instrument and provide rationale for making those changes.

Surveys and Questionnaires

The terms survey and questionnaire are often used interchangeably; however, there is a difference between the terms and you should not confuse the terms in your DNP project paper. Surveys are a measurement of attitudes, beliefs, and/or experiences of participants achieved by the asking of questions. In contrast, a questionnaire is a set of printed or written questions with a choice of answers.

Whether using surveys and/or questionnaires, you will need to provide detailed information about the use of each. Rationale will need to be given for the selection of the survey or questionnaire. Often there are various surveys and questionnaires that explore the same phenomenon (e.g., Grief Intensity Scale, Brief Grief Questionnaire, Inventory of Complicated Grief). It is critical that you provide rationale as to why you selected the specific surveys and questionnaires to use over other similar surveys and questionnaires.

You will need to describe previous populations for which the survey or questionnaire was used. The type of setting and method of delivery for prior survey and questionnaire use will also need to be described. The method of survey or questionnaire delivery may include face-to-face, telephone, mailing, or computer. The number of items on each survey or questionnaire should be mentioned, as well as the expected amount of time to complete each document. As discussed above, the reliability and validity of the survey or questionnaire instruments need to be identified.

It is likely that a cover letter will go out with a survey or questionnaire; you should place a copy of the cover letter in the appendices. In the project paper, you should clearly indicate how, where, how many times, and by whom potential participants were approached to complete a survey or questionnaire. The response rate to complete the survey or questionnaire must be identified and compared to the actual number of people who were approached. Differences in characteristics (e.g., age, gender, ethnicity) between those who opted to complete the survey or questionnaire and those who chose not to complete the documents should be identified. For example, note if elderly participants complete the survey or questionnaire at a higher rate than younger participants (Kelley, Clark, Brown, & Sitzia, 2003).

Observations

Quantitative *observation* is concerned with variables that are observed and recorded numerically (e.g., the number of times APRNs wash their hands during an 8-hour time period or the number of times patients are walked in the first 24 hours post-thoracotomy).

In a DNP project paper, the observer needs to be identified (e.g., DNP student, staff assistant) and the role of the observer needs to be clearly described. If there is more than one observer, you will need to describe how interrater-reliability was established. Interrater-reliability is the degree to which two or more raters or observers provide consistent estimates of the observed behavior. The tool for collecting observation data must be described and a copy of the tool should be placed in the appendix. Protocol for using the observation tool needs to be clearly outlined in the project paper.

Biophysiological and Physical Measurements

Many DNP project outcomes are evaluated through self-report and observation; however, a growing number of DNP students are using biophysiological and physical measurements. Biophysiological and physical phenomena (e.g., blood pressure, forced expiratory volume in 1 second) require specialized equipment and/or technology for measurement. You must describe, in detail, how the biophysiological and physical measurements were taken, who took the measurements, and the measurer's qualifications. For example, if the physical measurement is blood pressure, you need to discuss what size cuff was used, which arm was used, position of the participant, and whether a sphygmomanometer or blood pressure monitor was used and if the blood pressure was taken by licensed or unlicensed personnel.

Distinguish if the biophysiological and physical measurements are either in vivo or in vitro measures. In vivo measures are performed directly on or in participants and may be complex, such as renal arteriogram, or straightforward, such as an ear thermometer. In vitro measurements are performed outside the participant's body, such as blood analysis for electrolytes. You need to provide the rationale for why a particular biophysiological and/or physical measurement was selected and why. You should provide rationale if potential alternative measures were not used. Also, describe the specific training required to perform tests. Any associated costs for equipment or personnel must be indicated in the project paper.

Retrospective Chart Review

A retrospective chart review (RCR) is an important quantitative methodology, especially for QI projects. An RCR is a project design in which pre-recorded, patient-centered data are used to provide insights about patient care and/or evaluate healthcare outcomes (Worster & Haines, 2004). DNP students have no control over the accuracy of the medical records from which they will be abstracting data; therefore, RCRs are at risk for questionable validity. To enhance RCR validity, you must provide a meticulous and accurate description of the chart review protocol.

There are crucial points about RCR protocol to document. Begin with describing the phenomenon that was measured. For example, if you want to measure the rate at which nitroglycerin is administered for patient reports of angina in a cardiac care unit, prior to RCR, you will need to describe what qualifies as angina. Date parameters for the chart review need to be identified, and rationale for the date range should be provided. The number of charts reviewed must also be indicated and the rationale for the total charts reviewed must be provided. How you gained access to the charts for review should be described. Chart review tools are generally used to conduct RCRs. How the tools were developed needs to be described. Protecting patient confidentiality is a principal element in RCR and must be documented in the project paper.

Quantitative Data Collection Statement Example: The 16-item Relational Humility Scale (RHS; Davis et al., 2011) was used to assess humility in the clinic's APRNs. The RHS has 3 subscales: (1) Global Humility, (2), Superiority, and (3) Self-awareness. RHS items were completed using a 5-point Likert-like scale ranging from 1 = completely agree to 5 = completely disagree. Cronbach's alphas for full-scale score ranged from .90 to .95.

How you gained access to patient charts should be described. The RHS has demonstrated early evidence of construct validity because it correlates with empathy and forgiveness of an offender and positive relationship characteristics with a parent.

Qualitative Data Collection

Qualitative inquiry is concerned with human lived experiences (Schwandt, 2015); therefore, the purpose of qualitative data collection is to provide evidence for the lived experiences of patients (Polkinghorne, 2005). Interviews and focus groups are two of the most common types of data collection students use for DNP projects (Roush, 2019).

Interviews: Interviews are the most widely used approach for gathering qualitative data (Polkinghorne, 2005). Potter (1996) defined interviewing as a technique for gathering data from participants by asking questions and prompting them to respond verbally. Assisting participants to provide interview narratives is an activity that must be documented in the DNP project paper (Polkinghorne, 2005). Most qualitative interviews are dyadic. The interviewer knows in advance what experience they want the participant to share and therefore come to the interview with a format structure and predetermined questions. The three format structures are:

Structured: Generally, a structured format consists of a set of fixed questions that are administered verbally. There is minimal variation among questions and no scope for follow-up questions. Elaboration, on the participant's part, is unencouraged. Structured questions are useful for interviews that must be expedient, require limited depth from participants, and/or participant literacy is a concern (Gill, Stewart, Treasure, & Chadwick, 2008). Structured interviews are also used when a student has a well-developed understanding of the topic and a highly structured *questionnaire* that will provide participants with relevant and meaningful responses as options for the questions.

Semi-structured: Compared to structured interviews, semi-structured interviews are conversational and elicit in-depth narrative. Participants are encouraged, by the interviewer, to answer preset open-ended questions, which can be used in a flexible manner. The hallmark of a well-developed semi-structured interview ensures data are captured in key areas while allowing participants to bring their personality and perspective to the developing narrative. Preset questions are often referred to as an interview guide. Students need to indicate if the interview guide has been used before or if it was developed specifically for the current project. If the interview guide was previously used you should indicate on what populations and for what purposes it was used. If the interview guide was developed for the current project, students will need to explain their rationale for the questions selected. For example, was there a theoretical basis for developing the questions and/or were they based perhaps on a pilot study or on interview guides discussed in the literature.

Unstructured: Sometimes referred to as "discovery interviews," unstructured interviews are used when you do not have a predetermined view of the topic (Polit & Beck, 2019). For example, "What are information-seeking behaviors of community health nurses?" is a broad open-ended question that allows participants to freely explore their thought about the inquiry.

Irrespective of the selected qualitative interview format, you must document several key aspects of the interview in the DNP paper. Each of these aspects influence the participant's understandings and contributions to the final product. Proper documentation of these aspects in the methodology section will enhance the authenticity of the DNP paper.

Selection and rationale of the interview format: The chosen interview format needs to align with the purpose statement and/or PICOT question. For instance, if the purpose of the project is to learn steps intensive care unit nurses use to change central line dressings, a structured interview format will work best as a means to collect specific information in an efficient manner. It is critical that you identify, describe, and state the rationale for the selected interview format.

Recordings: If the interviews are being audio or video recorded, specific information must be included in the DNP project paper. For instance, the process for seeking the participants' permission to record must be described. When the recordings will be transcribed and by whom will need to be addressed. How the transcripts will be reviewed for accuracy will need to be included. Storage and/or destruction of the transcripts must be documented.

Developing the questions: How the interview questions were developed or selected must be included in the DNP paper. How the interviews were conducted (e.g., tape-recorded, note-taking), specific training the interviewer received, and technology used in conducting the interview must all be described.

Time allotment: Most dyad interviews are limited to one hour. Most one-hour interviews will not produce full and rich descriptions of the phenomenon being studied; therefore, two or more interviews may be required (Seidman, 2019). The time and number of interviews for each participant must be indicated. In addition, the rationale for the amount of time and number of interviews must be included.

Gaining access: The means for gaining access to participants need to be described. There are several methods used for gaining access to participants including recruiter databases, face-to-face recruitment, snowballing, and client lists. In addition to identifying the type of recruitment, you must fully explain the recruitment strategy and justification for the type of recruitment method selected.

Setting: The setting in which the interviews occurred will need to be described. If the interviews are online, you will need to indicate if they are synchronous or asynchronous. Any video online conferencing service that is used should be identified (e.g., Skype, BlueJeans).

Interviewer's presence: The interviewer's presence is a critical aspect of qualitative discovery (Mishler, 1996). How the interviewer listens, attends, and terminates the interview influences the participant's contributions and must be included in the DNP paper.

Skill acquisition: Qualitative interviewing has unique goals that require specialized skill sets (Polkinghorne, 2005). How the interviewer attained proper interviewing skills must be documented, including practice time and critique from knowledgeable interviewers.

Alternative explanations: The purpose of the interview is to provide alternative perspectives about the topic being studied. DNP students should not interview with the purpose of hoping to find support for their views about a particular phenomenon. Useful interviews describe unexpected and unanticipated accounts of an experience and must be fully described in the DNP paper.

Qualitative Data Collection Statement Example: Participants completed two questions that asked:

1. What aspect of culturally sensitive care is most important to you?
2. How can healthcare providers best address your care related to the aspect you selected?

Table 4.2

Trustworthiness in Qualitative Research

Criterion	Strategies to address in DNP Project Paper
Credibility: Students must convey to readers how they know the qualitative data is valid and accurate and that the original data has been credibly interpreted by students.	• Prolonged engagement • Persistent observation • Triangulation • Member check • Peer debriefing
Transferability: Students must demonstrate to readers that data are applicable to other settings and contexts.	• Thick, rich description
Confirmability and dependability: Students must convey to readers that data are based on the participants' perceptions and not the motivation or imagination of students.	• Audit trail
Dependability: Students must provide evidence that data would be replicated if interviews were connected with similar groups and in similar settings.	• Careful documentation and decision trail
Reflexivity: Students must provide information that they have examined their own assumptions, beliefs, and values and how this affected the interpretation of qualitative data.	• Diary

Source: Data from Lincoln, Y. S., & Guba, E. G. (1985). *Naturalistic Inquiry.* Newbury, CA: Sage.; Sim, J., & Sharp, K. (1998). A critical appraisal of the role of triangulation in nursing research. *International Journal of Nursing Studies, 35*(1–2), 23–31. doi:10.1016/s0020-7489(98)00014-5

Trustworthiness

As described earlier, DNP students who collect *quantitative* data must address the reliability and validity of the data assessment instruments or tools they use for measurement. DNP students who gather *qualitative* data must also address issues of reliability and validity. Because the collection of qualitative data does not involve the use of instruments or tools, the process of establishing reliability and validity is referred to as trustworthiness. Similar to reliability and validity, trustworthiness helps to establish if the qualitative findings can be trusted (Lincoln & Guba, 1985). The trustworthiness of qualitative data must be described in the DNP project paper and consists of four critical areas: (1) credibility, (2) transferability,

(3) dependability, and (4) confirmability. See Table 4.2 for definitions and strategies of each criterion for trustworthiness that need to be addressed in the DNP paper.

WRITING YOUR ANALYTIC PROCEDURES AND METHODS

It is helpful to remember that even the most experienced researchers are often challenged when it comes to analyzing quantitative and/or qualitative data. Seldom do quantitative and/or qualitative researchers work in isolation. It is only reasonable to assume that DNP students will need mentoring through the data analysis process. Early consultation with experienced faculty about analysis will likely be a wise investment of time and effort.

QUANTITATIVE ANALYSIS

Numerical data is transformed into useful information through the process of quantitative analysis. Students must communicate, in detail, the critical judgments and rationale used to make key decisions about the analysis of quantitative data. Listed below are several important steps that must be included in the project paper to enable readers to trust and understand the descriptions and explanations provided about the DNP project data.

1. An explanation of how the data were edited prior to analysis needs to be included. Students should describe the process they used for inspecting the data for completeness and accuracy. Students need to account for how they dealt with errors or misinformation. For example, a respondent may say in one question they have no history of heart disease but in another question indicate that they take digoxin and potassium supplements.
2. Data are often missing from questionnaires and surveys. Students need to explain how they handled missing data. For instance, if more than 10% of data is missing on a participant's survey, DNP students may decide to eliminate that survey from the project's analysis.
3. The coding and entering of data should be identified for readers. Coding is a quantification process of converting data into a numerical form (e.g., single = 1, married = 2).

4. Readers need to know if data were changed into a new format. For example, if a 7-point Likert Scale was reduced to a 5-point Likert Scale.

5. Students will want to identify if the data to be analyzed are:
   a. Univariate: contains only a single variable, such as age, gender, or height.
   b. Bivariate: data that consist of *two variables*, such as the relationship between age and the level of thyroid-stimulating hormone.
   c. Multivariate: data that represent *several variables*, such as the correlation between age, gender, steps walked postoperatively, and paralytic ileus.

6. Students will want to describe and provide rationale for the types of analyses that were conducted on the data, such as measures of central tendency, correlations, and multiple regression.

Quantitative Analysis Statement Example: Data from this project were cleaned and checked for outliers. Data were coded and transferred onto a data file via keyboard. Data were analyzed in SPSS Statistics for Windows, Version 23 (IBM, Armonk, NY). Calculations for descriptive statistics, including frequencies and percentages, were conducted for demographic variables.

QUALITATIVE ANALYSIS

Data analysis in qualitative research is a systematic process of searching and arranging the interview transcripts, observation notes, or other non-textual materials to increase the understanding of the phenomenon (Bogdan & Biklen, 2003). There are several key steps that must be reported as elements of qualitative analysis including data cleaning, chunking, coding, clustering, and making sense of the data for others. Each of these units of analysis must be carefully and fully described to enhance the rigor and trustworthiness of the DNP project.

Qualitative Analysis Statement Selection: Sense of belongingness was explored for LGBTQ patients seen at a primary healthcare clinic. Using constant comparison, transcripts were analyzed for theoretically relevant categories.

For Methods section review see Tables 4.3 and 4.4.

Table 4.3

Methods Section Checklist

Capturing the METHODS in IMRaD

The Methods section provides a detailed explanation of how the DNP project was conducted and the materials used in the process. Based on the methods section, other healthcare providers should be able to replicate the project and reproduce similar outcomes.

METHODS elements	Completed "Yes" or "No"	If "Yes," date completed: If "No," list steps needed to complete:
Project Design I have:		
• Described how the design supports the type(s) of data that will be needed.	_____	_____
• Included a compelling reason for why the selected design is best for this project.	_____	_____
• Provided rationale explaining the logical linkage between a selected design and the PICOT question and/or problem statement.	_____	_____
• Given sufficient detail so that another APRN could replicate the design for a similar project.	_____	_____
Context I have:		
• Indicated how context is defined for the project.	_____	_____
• Defined and discussed context based on the project's objectives?	_____	_____

(continued)

Table 4.3

Methods Section Checklist (*continued*)

METHODS elements	Completed "Yes" or "No"	If "Yes," date completed: If "No," list steps needed to complete:
Setting I have:		
• Identified types of services provided at the project's clinical or practice settings.	___	___
• Provided rationale for selecting the identified setting over other settings.	___	___
• Described how the setting may impact the project.		
Population and Sample I have:		
• Clearly distinguished the sample and setting in all sections of the paper.	___	___
• Described sample accessibility. Identified and described all sites from which the sample was selected.	___	___
• Formulated the exact number of participants.	___	___
• Provided a general description of relevant participant clinical and demographic variables.		
Sampling Plan I have:		

- Explained how the purposive sample was typical of population.
- Provided evidence that the convenience sample is not atypical of population.

Recruitment

I have:

- Identified rationale for the recruitment method.
- Described the use of incentives.
- Listed potential biases associated with the recruitment plan.
- Justified the sample size.

Ethical Considerations

I have:

- Secured IRB approval.
- Described steps taken to minimize participant risks.
- Supplied appropriate documentation of informed consent and consent letter in the appendices.

Implementation

I have:

- Described meetings with stakeholders who will be part of the project's implementation group, and included a description of frequency of meetings, organization of setting, role of participants who attended meetings, meeting agenda, and outcomes of meetings.
- Described potential barriers and facilitators to implementation.
- Outlined approval process for conducting implantation.

(continued)

Table 4.3

Methods Section Checklist (continued)

METHODS elements	Completed "Yes" or "No"	If "Yes," date completed: If "No," list steps needed to complete:
• Described project resources.	——	——
• Identified needed baseline data to evaluate outcomes.	——	——
• Discussed appropriate tainting for any interventions.		
Quantitative Data Collection I have:		
• Provided data to answer the PICOT question.	——	——
• Described congruency between conceptual and operational definitions.	——	——
• Indicated reliability and validity of instruments described.		
Qualitative Data Collection I have:		
• Described data collection strategies.	——	——
• Fully described the role of the student in data collection.	——	——
• Fully described the steps taken to assure accuracy of data.	——	——

Quantitative Analysis

I have:

- Presented the relevant results. _____
- Described the data analysis procedures. _____
- Ensured that the data help to answer the PICOT question. _____
- Determined if findings are supported by the literature review and theoretical framework. _____
- Described areas to establish trustworthiness. _____

Qualitative Analysis

I have:

- Assured the interpretive statements align with purpose of the DNP project. _____
- Indicated that inclusion and exclusion criteria were followed. _____
- Clearly defined concepts. _____
- Described logical relationships depicted among concepts. _____

IMRaD, Introduction, Methodology, Results, and Discussion; DNP, Doctor of Nursing Practice; IRB, Institutional Review Board

Table 4.4

Faculty Discussion Table

I have discussed the following Method sections with my faculty advisor:	Yes/No	Date discussed:
• Reasons a particular design was selected over other potential designs.	___	___
• Best possible sources of data to collect for the project (e.g., big data, simulation data).	___	___
• If technology is maximized to collect data.	___	___
• Academic timeline to be certain there is a reasonable alignment with the proposed design.	___	___
• How the selected design supports the validity, reliability, and/or trustworthiness of the project.	___	___
• Ways in which context will provide meaning to the project.	___	___
• Scope of the context. For example, should context be local or should it take on global dimensions?	___	___
• How might contextual implications influence data collection?	___	___
• How the organization's leadership style and philosophy may impact the project.	___	___
• How will the setting provide adequate data to match the project's objectives?	___	___
• Strengths and limitations of the setting and how those factors may impact a project.	___	___
• The setting's specific culture.	___	___
• If applicable, the setting's professional practice model.	___	___
• Appropriateness of the identified sample and the sample's linkage to a proposed project.	___	___
• Identified sample characteristics to be certain the characteristics are in agreement with inclusion and exclusion criteria for the DNP project.	___	___

- Potential participants and type of institutional review board (IRB) application.
- If the project's sample will best align with the project's objectives.
- How many participants are necessary for the project to demonstrate efficacy?
- Contingency plan if the recruitment method proves to be inadequate.
- Considering the sample, to whom can project results be generalized?
- Equitable selection of participants.
- Precautions for vulnerable populations.
- Plausible barriers and facilitators associated with the implementation.
- Strategize how to minimize identified barriers and maximize facilitators.
- A finalized version of the implementation protocol.
- Ideas for flyers, brochures, social media, and other options for recruitment.
- Reviewed the final version of all recruitment procedure.
- Begin an evaluation plan for the project.
- Determine if applicability of results is logical.
- Alignment of data collection strategies with project purpose.
- How to maximize the use of tables and graphics.
- Based on the data, if the interpretations and conclusions are realistic.

SUMMARY

The Methods section of the DNP project paper serves to explain the methodological approach, describe the methods of data collection, and describe the methods of analysis that were used. Students must justify these methodological choices and present an evaluation of the results of the decisions. A well-crafted Methods section, with attention to detail, will help portray a convincing image for the overall DNP project.

References

Agency for Healthcare Research and Quality. (2019). *Health information technology*. Retrieved from https://healthit.ahrq.gov/health-it-tools -and-resources/evaluation-resources/workflow-assessment-health-it -toolkit/all-workflow-tools/plan-do-check-act-cycle

Alexander, J. A., Weiner, B. J., & Griffith, J. (2006). Quality improvement and hospital financial performance. *Journal of Organizational Behavior, 27*(7), 1003–1029. doi:10.1002/job.401

Best, M., & Neuhauser, D. (2006). Walter A. Shewart 1924 and the Hawthorne factory. *Quality and Safety in Health Care, 15*(2), 142–143. doi:10.1136/qshc.2006.018093

Beyea, S. C., & Slattery, M. J. (2006). *Evidence-based practice in nursing: A guide to successful implementation*. Marblehead, MA: HCPro.

Black, K. (2010). *Business statistics: Contemporary decision making*. Hoboken, NJ: John Wiley & Sons.

Bogdan, R., & Biklen, S. K. (2003). *Qualitative research for education: An introduction to theory and methods*. Boston, MA: Allyn and Bacon.

Bonnel, B., & Smith, K. V. (2018). *Proposal writing for clinical nursing and DNP projects*. New York, NY: Springer Publishing Company.

Borrell, C., Espelt, A., Rodriquez-Sanz, M., & Navarro, V. (2007). Politics and health. *Journal of Epidemiology and Community Health, 61*(8), 658–659. doi:10.1136/jech.2006.059063

Davis, D. E., Hook, J. N., Worthington, E. L., Van Tongerson, D. R., Gartner, A. L., Jennings, D. J., & Emmons, R. A. (2011). Relational humility: Conceptualization and measuring humility as a personality judgment. *Journal of Personality Assessment, 93*, 225–234. doi:10 .1080/00223891.2011.558871

Drennan, J., Duffield, C., Scott, A. P., Ball, J., Brady, N. M., Murphy, A., . . . Griffiths, P. (2018). A protocol to measure the impact of intentional changes to skill-mix in medical and surgical wards. *Journal of Advanced Nursing, 74*, 2912–2921. doi:10.1111/jan.13796

Fineout-Overholt, E., Melnyk, B. M., & Schultz, A. (2005). Transforming healthcare from inside out: Advancing evidence-based practice in the 21st century. *Journal of Professional Nursing, 21*(6), 335–344. doi:10.1016/j.profnurs.2005.10.005

Freeman, R. E. (1984). *Strategic management: A stakeholder approach*. Boston, MA: Pitman.

Gill, P., Stewart, K., Treasure, E., & Chadwick, B. (2008). Methods of data collection in qualitative research: Interviews and focus groups. *British Dental Journal, 204*(6), 291–295.

Glassman, K. S. (2017). Using data in nursing practice. *American Nurse Today, 12*(11), 45–47.

Gray, J. R., Groves, S. K., & Sutherland, S. (2017) *Burns and Grove's: The practice of nursing research: Appraisal synthesis, and generation of evidence*. Philadelphia, PA: Elsevier.

Harvey, G., & Kitson, A. (2016). PARIHS revisited: From heuristic to integrated framework for the successful implementation of knowledge into practice. *Implementation Science, 11*(1), 33. doi:10.1186/s13012-016-0398-2

Hawe, P., Shiell, A., Riley, T., & Gold, L. (2004). Methods for exploring implementation and local context within a cluster randomized community intervention trial. *Journal of Epidemiology and Community Health, 58*(9), 788–793. doi:10.1136/jech.2003.014415

Herek, G. M., & Garnets, L. D. (2007). Sexual orientation and mental health. *Annual Review of Clinical Psychology, 3*, 353–375. doi:10.1146/annurev.clinpsy.3.022806.091510

Institute for Healthcare Improvement. (2019). *IHI triple aim*. Retrieved from http://www.ihi.org/engage/initiatives/tripleaim/pages/default.aspx

Jager, J., Putnick, D. L., & Bornstein, M. H. (2017). More than just convenient: The scientific merits of homogeneous convenience samples. *Monographs of the Society for Research in Child Development, 82*(2), 13–30. doi:10.1111/mono.12296

Kallet, R. H. (2004). How to write the methods section of a research paper. *Respiratory Care, 49*(10), 1229–1232.

Kelley, K., Clark, B., Brown, V., & Sitzia, J. (2003). Good practice in the conduct and reporting of survey research. *International Journal of Quality in Health Care, 15*(3), 261–266. doi:10.1093/intqhc/mzg031

Lincoln, Y. S., & Guba, E. G. (1985). *Naturalistic inquiry*. Newbury, CA: Sage.

Mishler, E. G. (1996). *Research interviewing: Context and narrative*. Cambridge, MA: Harvard University Press.

Mosadeghrad, A. M. (2014). Factors affecting medical service quality. *Iranian Journal of Public Health, 43*(2), 210–220.

Newhouse, R. P., Dearholt, S. L., Poe, S. S., Pugh, L. C., & White, K. M. (2005). Evidence-based practice: A practical approach to implementation. *Journal of Nursing Administration, 35*(1), 35–40. doi:10.1097/00005110-200501000-00013

Polit, D. F., & Beck, C. T. (2019). *Essentials of nursing research: Appraising evidence for nursing practice*. Philadelphia, PA: Wolters Kluwer Health/Lippincott Williams & Wilkins.

Polkinghorne, D. E. (2005). Language and meaning: Data collection in qualitative research. *Journal of Counseling Psychology, 32*(2), 137–145. doi:10.1037/0022-0167.52.2.137

Potter, W. J. (1996). *An analysis of thinking and research about qualitative methods*. Mahwah, NJ: Erlbaum.

Rapport, F., Clay-Williams, R., Churruca, K., Shih, P., Hogden, A., & Braithwaite, J. (2018). The struggle of translating science into action: Foundational concepts of implementation science. *Journal of Evaluation in Clinical Practice, 24*, 117–126. doi:10.1111/jep.12741

Riley, W. J., Moran, J. W., Corso, L. C., Beitsch, L. M., Bialek, R., & Cofsky, A. (2010). Defining quality improvement in public health. *Journal of Public Health Management and Practice, 16*(1), 5–7. doi:10.1097/PHH.0b013e3181bedb49

Roush, K. (2019). *A nurse's step-by-step guide to writing a dissertation or scholarly project*. New York, NY: Springer Publishing Company.

Rudisill, F., & Druley, S. (2004). Which Six Sigma metric should I use? *Quality Progress, 37*(3), 104.

Schwandt, T. A. (2015). *The sage dictionary of qualitative inquiry*. Thousand Oaks, CA: Sage.

Seidman, I. E. (2019). *Interviewing as qualitative research. A guide for researchers in education and the social sciences*. New York, NY: Teachers College Press.

Sim, J., & Sharp, K. (1998). A critical appraisal of the role of triangulation in nursing research. *International Journal of Nursing Studies, 35*(1–2), 23–31. doi:10.1016/s0020-7489(98)00014-5

Stevens, K. R. (2004). *ACR Star model of EBP: Knowledge transformation*. San Antonio, TX: Academic Center for Evidence-Based Practice, The University of Texas Health Science Center at San Antonio. Retrieved from http://www.acestar.utcssa.edu

Titler, M. G., Kleiber, C., Steelman, V. J., Rakel, B. A., Budreau, G., Everett, L. Q., . . . Goode, C. J. (2001). The Iowa model to promote evidence-based practice to promote quality care. *Critical Care Nursing Clinics of North America, 13*(4), 497–509.

Tomoaia-Cotisel, A., Scammon, D. L., Waitzman, N. J., Cronholm, P. J., Halladay, J. R., Driscoll, D. L., . . . Stange, K. C. (2013). Context matters: The experience of 14 research teams in systematically reporting contextual factors important for practice change. *Annals of Family Medicine, 11*(Suppl. 1), S115–S123. doi:10.1370/afm.1549

White, K. M., Dudley-Brown, S., & Terhaar, M. F. (2019). *Translation of evidence into nursing and health care*. New York, NY: Springer Publishing Company.

Williams, B. (2015). Understanding qualitative research. *American Nurse Today, 10*(7), 40–42.

Williams, H. K. (1919). Religious Education, The Group Plan. *The Biblical World, 53*(1), 78–81.

Worster, A., & Haines, T. (2004). Advanced statistics: Understanding medical record review (MRR) studies. *Academic Emergency Medicine, 11*(2), 187–192.

5

IMRaD: Results Content for a DNP Project Paper

After reading this chapter, learners should be able to:

1. Build a demographic table.
2. Calculate a response rate.
3. Identify key element elements of quantitative and qualitative analysis report.
4. Differentiate between tables and graphs.

INTRODUCTION

"Realists do not fear the results of their study" (Dostoevsky, 1821–1881). Students and experienced academics, at times, hold expectations for a project's results that may not emerge. Untoward or unexpected project results should not be feared or viewed as failures. In fact, much is learned and gained from unanticipated project results. To advance healthcare and patient outcomes, project results must be presented wholly and with integrity. Results should not be misleadingly manipulated to align with project objectives. Instead, meaningful and thoughtful explanations should be presented to illuminate any misalignment between project objectives and results.

The purpose of a Results section is to clearly, credibly, and logically state the findings of the Doctor of Nursing Practice (DNP) project. It may seem an oversimplification to state that a Results section should include only findings; however, some novice and experienced authors attempt to include far-reaching generalizations in a Results section.

REPORTING RESULTS

Interpretations of findings are reviewed in the Discussion Section. Similar to a Methods section, the final draft of a Results section is written in the past tense. To help readers refocus on the central theme of your project, begin the Results section by concisely restating the project's purpose.

There are four necessary components to include in a Results section: (1) response rate, (2) sample size, (3) demographics, and (4) findings. Prior to discussing these components, open the Results section with a short paragraph that informs readers of the areas to be described. For example, "The Results section presents findings from the numeric analyses as well as interpretations of patient responses to semi-structured questions. Demographic and clinical variables are presented with emphasis on relevant findings."

RESPONSE RATES

Response rate and completion rate provide readers with valuable insights about the thoroughness of data collection. Response rate and completion rate are sometimes used interchangeably. However, there is a difference between the two terms that should be noted in your project paper. Response rate denotes the number of project participants who completed project surveys divided by the number of participants who made up the entire sample group. For example:

100 email surveys sent to potential participants
Number of participants who entered the survey: 75
Number of participants who completed the survey: 50
Response rate: Number of completed surveys/Number of emails sent
Response rate = 50%

Completion rate designates the number of surveys completed and returned divided by the number of surveys initiated by participants. Only participants who have initiated the survey are included in the completion rate, and only participants who completed the full survey can increase the completion rate statistic. For example:

100 email surveys sent to potential participants
Number of participants who entered the survey: 75
Number of participants who completed the survey: 50
Completion rate = Number of completed surveys/Number of participants who entered the survey
Completion rate = 66%

Whether a response rate, a completion rate, or both are reported, it is important to describe in the project paper how the rate(s) was calculated.

Describing Ways to Increase Response Rates

It is important to describe any factors that enabled achievement of a satisfactory response rate. For example, include information about the survey design. Let readers know what was done to make the survey unambiguous and easy to understand. For instance, what grade level was the survey written for? Did content and/or survey experts review the survey before distribution? Indicate if the survey was pilot tested on a small sample before distribution to the project's participants. Describe how long, on average, it took pilot participants to complete surveys. Surveys should take 5 minutes or fewer to complete. Surveys that require more than 10 minutes to complete will likely result in a lower response rate. Describe any problems participants may have encountered in the pilot survey and all steps taken to correct any problems.

Participants generally like to have a sense of buy-in with the project. A way to increase a sense of buy-in participation is to provide survey results to participants. In qualitative research, member checking is a way to enhance the project's credibility and improve participation. Participant incentives, described in the Methods section, are also a way to increase participation.

Sending tactful reminders to participants is a critical means of increasing participation. Be certain to describe how many reminders were sent and when they were sent. Usually no more than two reminders are sent, and the time of day and day of week the reminders were sent need to be changed to maximize the number of participants reached. A copy of follow-up reminders should be placed in the paper's appendix. If used, each tactic to increase participation needs to be described in the project paper.

Describing Low Response and Completion Rates

Typically, surveys or sections of surveys have lower than anticipated response rates. In the project paper, it is important to describe possible reasons for low response rates and solutions used to correct problems associated with low response rates. For example, *incomplete data* is a fairly common low completion rate problem. Incomplete data indicates that participants are not providing the information needed. In the project paper, indicate possible reasons a particular question was not answered as frequently as other questions (e.g., participant fatigue, sensitive question) and what was done to address the low completion rate problem (e.g., rewrote question, removed question). It is important to note in the paper if participants who completed a survey were in some way different from those who did not complete a survey (e.g., age, gender, geographic location). In addition, describe any adjustments made to a survey based on less-than-anticipated early response rates.

SAMPLE SIZE AND DEMOGRAPHICS

Sample size defines the number of participants who were recruited and agreed to participate in the project (Gray, Groves, & Sutherland, 2017). In the paper, state the final sample size and identify any subgroups. A subgroup is a subset of participants who share a common characteristic, such as age or income range. Reporting the number of participants in the project will help readers estimate the validity and generalizability of findings. Report the sample size next to an italicized "*n*," which is the statistical abbreviation for sample size. For example, $n = 20$ indicates there were 20 participants in the project. Although it was reported in the Methods section how the sample is to be obtained, also report in the Results section how the sample was actually obtained. For example, "Convenience sampling was used as the sampling method."

The term demography comes from Greek means "description of the people." Demographics are characteristics (e.g., age, gender, income) of participants who were assessed during the project and used to describe the sample. Demographics should be reported in the aggregate for each characteristic or attribute. Demographic information should not be listed for each participant (Roush, 2019). Report only the demographics that are central to the purpose of the project and are germane to the problem statement and/or PICOT question.

Demographic variables are obtained from the demographic sheet that participants complete at the beginning of data collection. When the project is complete, demographic variables are analyzed to create a profile of the sample, which may be referred to in the paper as *sample characteristics*. Sample characteristics are generally presented in table and narrative form.

In addition to providing readers with an overall profile of the sample, indicate in the narrative any trends that demographic data suggest. For example, the number of immigrant participants in the sample may reflect the immigrant share in the general population. Describe any correlations (i.e., the degree to which two or more variables are systematically related) detected in the demographic data. For instance, millennial participant's may be more educated than other age groups in the sample. In addition, describe any combination of demographic variables that illuminate a concept or phenomenon, such as that more Americans are living in multigenerational homes, and young adults are edging out older adults as the most likely group to live in multigenerational homes. Clinical variables (e.g., blood pressure, body mass index, hematocrit) are as important as demographic variables. Report key clinical variables along with demographic variables.

The following demographic variables are frequently reported in DNP project papers:

- **Age (or birth date)**: Age is one of the most common demographic questions asked on surveys. In the narrative, describe how age-related demographic questions may elicit different responses in relation to certain topics. For example, survey questions about chronic care health insurance plans will likely be answered differently by respondents in their 20s compared with respondents in their 70s.
- **Ethnicity**: Answers to ethnicity or cultural questions may impact how other survey questions are answered and, therefore, can be described in the narrative. For example, a question about environment may have markedly different answers by Native American respondents raised in rural

Arizona compared with Latino respondents raised in Manhattan.

- **Gender and sex**: In the narrative, use gender as a cultural term (e.g., social roles, personal identification) when referring to men and women as groups. Use the term sex when making biological distinctions (e.g., secondary sex characteristics).
- **Level of education**: Depending on the topic and survey question, level of education can often leverage responses. Variation in responses, associated with level of education, should be noted in the narrative. A respondent's level of education can often uncover unique findings.
- **Professional or employment status**: In the narrative, factor in respondents' experiences or biases related to profession or employment. For example, a financial planner may answer questions about money management differently than a daycare worker. Unemployed respondents may have significantly different responses to a survey than employed respondents; therefore, comparisons should be described in the narrative.

Clearly, collecting demographic data will help readers better understand factors that possibly influence respondents' survey answers. Demographic information is invaluable in helping cross-tabulate to compare sub-groups in a sample. In addition, demographic data aid in examining how respondents' answers vary among groups within a sample, and similar samples, described in the literature. The components and design of the demographic table will depend, in part, on the topic and project sample. Descriptive statistics (e.g., mean, median, mode) are generally used to describe demographic and clinical variables. Table 5.1 is an example of a demographic table.

FINDINGS

The purpose of the findings component of a Results section is to summarize primary conclusions about the DNP project.

Fast Facts

Findings in a Results section must be presented in a logical sequence.

Table 5.1

Example of a Table for Sociodemographic Characteristics of DNP Project Participants (n = 100)

Characteristic	n = 100
Age (years):	
≤ 20	9 (9)
21–30	8 (8)
31–40	17 (17)
41–50	42 (42)
≥ 51	24 (24)
Minimum–maximum	18–(83)
Median IQR	
Sexual Orientation (optional; choose all that apply):	
__ asexual	2 (2%)
__ bisexual	5 (5%)
__ gay	8 (8%)
__ straight (heterosexual)	64 (64%)
__ lesbian	9 (9%)
__ pansexual	1 (1%)
__ queer	2 (2%)
__ questioning or unsure	3 (3%)
__ an identity not listed: please specify _____	0 (0%)
__ prefer not to disclose	4 (4%)
Highest level of education:	
Primary	4 (4%)
Secondary	18 (18%)
University (undergraduate)	78 (78%)
Occupation:	
Student	14 (14%)
Employed	79 (79%)
Unemployed	7 (7%)
Marital Status:	
Single	42 (42%)
In a relationship/partnered	14 (14%)
Married	46 (46%)

DNP, Doctor of Nursing Practice

Findings may be presented logically in the following ways: (1) in order of a project's timeline, (2) in order of the project objectives or aims, and (3) in the order of test analyses presented in the Methods section. The logical sequence of findings in a Results section will establish the order of summary in the forthcoming Discussion section. Findings in a Results section are presented as quantitative and/or qualitative reports, depending on the methodologies used for data collection. The following is a discussion about formatting findings for projects in which quantitative analysis is used.

Presentation of Quantitative Analysis

It is appropriate to begin the project's discussion of quantitative findings with a review of the statistical tests used to analyze project data. The statistical software packages and spreadsheets will provide voluminous quantities of data analysis about the project's findings. It is up to the DNP student and advisors, to determine what analyses should be presented as part of the current project and which analyses should be saved for future articles or reports. Selecting the findings to present requires critical thinking.

Fast Facts

Findings that best answer a PICOT question or illuminate aims or objectives will need to be presented in the project paper.

Discussion about statistical tests used should include important pieces of information:

- *The name of the statistical test.* Because statistical tests are specifically designed to answer certain questions, it is important to provide the rationale for using each identified test. A statistician is often a beneficial resource to provide needed statistical rationale.
- *The reported value of the tabulated statistic.* The numeric value of the statistic will enable readers to better interpret the meaning of the results.
- *The significance.* Significance is the degree to which a finding is reliable and reproducible. To differentiate from clinical significance, the significance for research findings is stated as *statistically significant* (Vogt & Johnson, 2016).

- *Level of significance.* The level of significance is the probability that an analysis result will be produced by chance alone rather than by the effects of an intervention. In the project paper, the level of significance will be stated as a probability. The probability is abbreviated as p and is followed by a number, e.g., $p < .05$ or $p < .01$ (Vogt & Johnson, 2016).

In the text, write a systematic description of the analyzed results. It is important to highlight for readers any findings that are relevant to the PICOT question or project objectives. Remember, at this juncture, the purpose is only to point out the findings; interpretation and discussion of findings will occur in the next section of the paper.

Fast Facts

Avoid using the word "prove" in the text. Analysis results cannot prove anything but may provide evidence to support the project's aims or objectives.

In the text, avoid describing data that is not relevant to your topic. A Results section narrative for quantitative analysis is easily laden with discussion of numbers, which readers generally find wearisome. To avoid reader fatigue and enliven the presentation of findings, a narrative is often accompanied with well-planned charts and graphs (Polit & Beck, 2019).

Most quantitative analysis sections will include non-narrative elements, such as tables and figures. Non-narrative elements should be a concise and easily understandable way to present large amounts of, often multifaceted, data. It is critical to remember that statistical data reported in the narrative should not overlap or be repeated in the non-narrative elements.

Tables are compilations of data in the form of columns and rows. Figures may include drawings, such as charts, graphs, and illustrations. Each table and figure must have an accurate heading and title. In the text, refer to the table or figure by number. For instance, "As demonstrated in Figure 10, patients at clinic A had lower medication adherence rates than patients at clinic B." All tables and figures must be numbered consecutively.

Almost invariably, some of the project findings will fail to support the outcome objectives. Be sure to document negative findings in the Results section. The upcoming Discussion section will provide plausible explanations of why the negative results may have occurred.

Presentation of Qualitative Analysis

Depending on the type of qualitative method (e.g., case study, phenomenological, ethnographic, grounded theory), there are various methods of analysis that may be used. It is important, regardless of the research method used, to carefully report each step that was taken in the analysis of qualitative data. The following are areas to address in the project paper about qualitative analysis and will be applicable to most types of qualitative studies.

- Identify the type of qualitative method used, and provide the rationale for why the method was appropriate for your project.
- Identify the type of qualitative analysis method:
  - Thematic analysis
  - Grounded theory
  - Interpretive phenomenological analysis
  - Discourse analysis
  - Narrative analysis
- Identify the sampling process.
- Describe how the data saturation point was reached.
- Provide insight on how you became familiar with the context.
- Explain how the data analysis was organized and prepared.
- Indicate how the potential for bias was handled.
- Describe, in detail, the coding process used.
- Describe the process of how categories or themes were formed from the data.
- Describe commonalities and divergences among the categories.
- Include verbatim participant quotations to illuminate the main themes that emerged. Be judicious in the use of quotations to prevent the project paper from becoming too long and tedious to read.
- Include contradictions and inconsistencies that may have occurred in participants' data. A primary purpose of qualitative work is to show divergent views of social and healthcare phenomena.
- Interpretive analyses must be presented with transparency so that readers may follow the logical process used to reach conclusions about the data.

Refer to Tables 5.2 and 5.3 for review of Results section.

Table 5.2

Results Section Checklist

Capturing the METHODS in IMRaD

A Results section is an unbiased presentation of a project's findings based on the methodologies used to collect data. Project findings are arranged in a logical sequence without interpretation.

Results elements I have:	Completed "Yes" or "No"	If "Yes," date completed: If "No," list steps needed to complete:
• Logically organized the statistical findings.		
• Reported the sample size.		
• Calculated and reported the response rate.		
• Documented relevant demographic and clinical variables.		
• Provided a narrative description of the sample.		
• Labeled and numbered all tables and graphs appropriately.		
• Provided the analyses results with no interpretation of results.		
• Checked with certainty that tables and graphs do not repeat information in the narrative.		
• Addressed each project objective in the analysis.		

IMRaD, introduction, methodology, results, and discussion

Table 5.3

Faculty Discussion Topics

I have discussed the following Results sections with my faculty advisor:	Yes/No	Date discussed:
• Level of measurement (e.g., nominal, ordinal, interval, ratio) for each statistical analysis.	___	___
• Identification of themes for qualitative sections.	___	___
• Selection of appropriate statistical tests.	___	___
• Verifies key findings are present.	___	___
• Strategies for reporting negative results.	___	___

SUMMARY

The Results section should be a clear and objective presentation of the project's findings. Key findings are presented in both narrative and non-narrative forms. Key findings are presented as the totality of project outcomes. Discussion, conclusions, and recommendations will be presented in the Discussion section.

References

Gray, J. R., Groves, S. K., & Sutherland, S. (2017). *Burns and Grove's: The practice of nursing research: Appraisal synthesis, and generation of evidence*. Philadelphia, PA: Elsevier.

Polit, D. F., & Beck, C. T. (2019). *Essentials of nursing research: Appraising evidence for nursing practice*. Philadelphia, PA: Wolters Kluwer Health/Lippincott Williams & Wilkins.

Roush, K. (2019). *A nurse's step-by-step guide to writing a dissertation or scholarly project*. New York, NY: Springer Publishing Company.

Vogt, W. P., & Johnson, R. B. (2016). *The Sage dictionary of statistics and methodology: A nontechnical guide for the social sciences*. Los Angeles, CA: Sage.

6

IMRa<u>D</u>: Discussion Content for a DNP Project Paper

After reading this chapter, learners should be able to:

1. Prepare a written discussion of quantitative and/or qualitative results.
2. Describe types of project limitations.
3. Explain how to detect bias in a project's data.

INTRODUCTION

The Discussion section is considered one of the most critical components of a Doctor of Nursing Practice (DNP) project paper. Broadly, the purpose of general discussion is to reach decisions and share ideas. Similarly, the purpose of a Discussion section in a DNP paper is to draw conclusions about project findings and share ways the project's outcomes may be applied to clinical practice (Roush, 2019). In a Discussion section, DNP students interpret the significance of their projects in light of the findings in the Results sections. A Discussion section is generally composed of five primary elements: (1) explanation of results (i.e., key findings, outcomes), (2) references to previous research and evidence, (3) deduction, (4) limitations, and (5) conclusions.

As with other project paper sections, begin the Discussion section with a brief review of the project purpose and ideas to be covered in the current section. For example, "In this project, a relaxation meditation model was implemented for elderly (≥ 65 years) residents in a long-term care facility. This section will provide an understanding of facilitators and barriers of initiating a relaxation meditation model for elderly residents." This brief overview may help remind readers of the problem outlined in the Introduction section. Do not self-plagiarize (Joyner, Rouse, & Glatthorn, 2013). Instead, write a synthesis and summary of the problem from the introductory statement and literature review. Be consistent in using the same variables, concepts, and key terms used in the previous Introduction, Methods, and Results sections.

EXPLANATION OF RESULTS

It may be helpful to think of a discussion section as an inverted pyramid. For example, organize the Discussion section from the general to the specific while describing project outcomes and their linkages to literature, theory, and, importantly for DNP projects, clinical practice. Begin by succinctly restating the problem statement and/or objectives addressed in the DNP project's Introduction section. Briefly summarize the findings to provide answers or discussion for each problem or objective. Develop a clear and succinct statement, no more than one paragraph, for each primary result. Examples of how to begin opening statements include:

- The outcome of objective one indicates…
- Answers to the PICOT question demonstrate a correlation among…
- The survey analysis confirms…
- In line with the PICOT question…
- Contrary to the proposed aim of the project…
- The results contradict the claim that…
- The results in this project suggest…. However, based on findings in similar projects, a more plausible explanation might be…

At this point, it is critical to remember that a brief summary of findings is expected but data from the Results section must not be restated.

Fast Facts

It is important that the Discussion section takes the form of commentary instead of repeating statistical and/or narrative results.

If results must be presented in the Discussion section, care must be taken that they are summarized in the context of current literature and not presented as a review of the Results section. For example, "In Table 2, a significant ($p \leq .05$) correlation was presented for the relationship between nurse manager leadership style and staff attrition." is a restatement of results. Instead, an improved statement for the Discussion section may be "Consistent with results of previous studies, results in this project demonstrated a positive correlation between leadership style and staff retention." The literature used for establishing context must be from peer-reviewed, top-tier journals in nursing or other professions. To keep the discussion current, it is expected that literature published within the last three years be used. Conclusions that are drawn from the project findings need to be accurate and non-contrived.

Be certain that explanations for the findings relate to the expectations of the objectives and to the literature reviewed in the Introduction section. Clearly explain why the findings are acceptable in relation to the project and how the findings fit seamlessly with published scholarly works and research. Remember to provide a reference for all studies mentioned in the project paper. When discussing findings, indicate if the results were expected and provide an explanation for each expected result. It is important to inform readers of any trends or patterns that emerged from the findings and offer explanations for those findings. In presenting the findings, it is important to discuss both statistically significant results and non-statistically significant results. Readers will want to know about patterns, principles, and key relationships among the significant and non-significant findings.

It is important to remember that while the results may seem obvious to a student, to less-informed readers results are not always transparent and easily understandable. To help provide clarity for readers, structure discussion of interpretations using these approaches:

- Highlight correlations found in surveys, questionnaires, or other forms of quantitative data.
- Discuss patterns or relationships found among project outcomes.
- Contextualize the results with the theoretical framework described in the Introduction section.
- Provide rationale for unexpected results and evaluate the significance of those results.
- Describe alternative explanations for results and develop an argument to support the explanations.

A rich Discussion section includes analysis and evaluation of any unexpected findings. Depth of discussion will be needed to explain unforeseen findings. Begin with a description of the unanticipated finding. Follow the description with an interpretation of why the unexpected finding may have appeared and its potential significance to the overall project. In some projects, more than one unexpected finding may occur. Describe unexpected findings in the order they appeared in the analysis of data section.

In addition to unexpected findings, sometimes a Results section may suggest that a DNP project's clinical intervention or practice changes proffered unwarranted outcomes. Untoward outcomes do not warrant a Discussion section that interprets the DNP project as a failure. Reviewed literature and robust theoretical underpinnings may strongly indicate that a clinical or systems intervention is fail-safe. However, organizations and their participants may unintentionally, or occasionally with intention, alter seemingly predictable DNP project outcomes. This is not a time to accept defeat. In fact, there is much to learn from when interventions do not work and particularly why they did not work. Providing readers with an understanding of unanticipated intervention outcomes is a critical component of a Discussion section.

In the Methods and Results sections, emphasis was placed on the sample and related demographic and clinical variables. A distinct discussion of the sample is warranted in the Discussion section (Polit & Beck, 2019). Discrepancies in the sample and broader population will need to be identified and described in the paper. For example, a project's population is predominantly college-educated and the sample is composed of participants without a high school diploma. Conceivable explanations for the inconsistency will need to be provided. A discussion about inconvenient findings must include in-depth comparing and contrasting with other projects and studies used to support the DNP project. Careful comparing and contrasting of literature may help determine factors that influenced negative results. Factors may include variations in populations, samples, organizational cultures, and settings. Other factors may include:

- Variations in patient acuity and disease chronicity.
- Unexpected organizational participant attrition.
- Unforeseen resource restriction.
- Reversal of key stakeholder support.
- Unaccounted characteristics of project participants.

The theoretical framework discussed in the Introduction section will need to be revisited in light of findings in the Results section. Some students accomplish this with a separate discussion of one to two paragraphs about how project results support the use of a theoretical framework. Other students may organize the entire discussion of findings within the context or structure of the theoretical framework. Some students may choose to assimilate statements about how select findings align with the theoretical framework throughout the discussion section of their papers.

In conclusion, remember to avoid overinterpretation of results. Interpretation contains a great deal of subjectivity and it is easy to create wide-ranging generalizations with the data. Refrain from reading more into the findings than is there. In the final analysis, the data, whether numeric or narrative, are only data and are dependent on a transparent and frank interpretation. The length of the Discussion section should not exceed the length of the other Introduction, Methodology, Results, and Discussion (IMRaD) sections combined. The explanation of results needs to conclude with a concise summary of the key findings. See Box 6.1 for key phrases used in writing a findings section.

BOX 6.1 KEY PHRASES FOR FINDINGS

- From the review, key themes emerge, including...
- This is a critical finding in the exploration of...
- This project confirmed the use of...
- The primary result demonstrates...
- The analysis of evidence to supports...
- Based on the project's results it is evident that...
- Planned comparisons between interventions found that...

REFERENCES TO PREVIOUS RESEARCH AND EVIDENCE

Remember, there is no DNP project that is so novel or restricted in focus that it has no meaningful relation to published evidence and/or research. Comparing and contrasting findings to other published works supports the importance of the current DNP paper's findings and it will emphasize in what ways the current findings make a unique contribution to clinical practice. See Box 6.2 for key phrases used in writing references to previous studies.

Fast Facts

A key feature of a Discussion section is to show how findings fit relative to the existing body of knowledge about the project's topic.

BOX 6.2 KEY PHRASES FOR REFERENCES TO OTHER STUDIES

- Others have demonstrated that… enhances…
- Results from other projects are in alignment with…
- Similar project conclusions were reached by…
- The results of this project are consistent with…
- The findings in this project are in accordance with…
- The results correlate well with the work of…
- In comparing the results of this project with other projects, it must be pointed out that…

DEDUCTION

Deduction in a DNP project paper describes how project results may be applied more generally to clinical and healthcare systems initiatives. Often, best practices emerge from the knowledge gained in DNP projects. It is this knowledge that may be applied more broadly to improve clinical circumstances. See Box 6.3 for key phrases used in writing deduction statements.

BOX 6.3 KEY PHRASES FOR DEDUCTION STATEMENTS

- The findings support the idea that…
- Results demonstrate that…is not always true.
- The findings are related to…
- A difference between these findings is attributed to…
- The findings support that it is justified to…

LIMITATIONS

DNP students are recognized for being deeply committed to optimizing patient care quality and generally do everything possible to assure a faultless DNP project. However, no DNP project is perfect and project limitations are to be expected. All DNP projects require a discussion of limitations. The limitations discussion is not an opportunity to provide excuses for project weaknesses. The limitations section is, however, an opportunity to identify project limitations and describe how they may have impacted project results. An objective tone is used to describe limitations.

The limitations of a DNP project are characteristics of methodology, design, and/or theory that may have unduly influenced a project's findings. Limitations may place constraints on transferability or generalizability of project findings to clinical practice. The utility of findings may be impaired by limitations and thus must be scrupulously discussed. It is far better for a student to identify and claim a project's limitations than to have the limitations later pointed out by faculty advisors or other discerning readers.

Fast Facts

Discussing a project's limitations has many benefits.

Discussion of limitations provides an opportunity to make recommendations for further practice initiatives and collaborative research projects. A DNP project's limitations can provide a way for unanswered healthcare questions to become more focused and amenable for future research. Forthright admission of a project's limitations enables students to demonstrate they have thought judiciously and critically about their projects, comprehended relevant literature, and systematically evaluated methodologies used to conduct DNP projects. Discussing a project's limitations requires more than identifying obvious weaknesses, such as "a convenience sample was used." Listing only obvious limitations may leave readers speculating about limitations that were intentionally omitted. Instead, put forth limitations that are derived from critical analysis of a project's theory and methodologies that result from critical reflection of the overall project.

Potential Methodological Limitations

Sample size: DNP students do not have unlimited time to recruit participants. In addition, real-life clinical settings may lack sufficient numbers of participants to enroll in a project. If a sample size is inadequate, students may be overly challenged to cull significant relationships from project data. Large sample sizes are often needed to demonstrate significant correlations among variables in surveys and questionnaires. If a sample size is inadequate, it is difficult to generalize (quantitative data) or transfer (qualitative data) findings to similar groups. Reasons for inadequate sample sizes need to be described in the project paper.

Insufficient data: Lack of data or unreliable data will impair the scope of quantitative and qualitative analysis. Insufficient data may prevent discovering meaningful relationships or trends among project variables. These limitations must be described in the paper. Students will need to provide plausible explanations for data that are missing or not reliable. This is not a reason to despair; inadequate data can be a sound reason for recommending future projects.

Lack of prior research and/or evidence literature: The success of a Discussion section is dependent on citing relevant research or evidence to form a deeper understanding of a DNP project's results. Much of the Discussion section literature was likely referenced in the introductory section and literature review. If, for any reason, there does not seem to be adequate literature to support additional insights and understandings into a project's outcomes, consult with a health sciences reference librarian. A limitation of previous evidence can form the basis for an opportunity to discuss the need for future projects and research endeavors.

Measurement issues: It seems, more often than not, that clinicians and researchers wish they had gathered additional data once they begin the interpretation of findings. In retrospect, it is always easy to see how additional survey questions could have addressed a particular problem at a deeper or more meaningful level. It is important to acknowledge any measurement issues in the Discussion section and make recommendations for future projects and/or research.

Issues in self-reporting: A primary advantage of self-report data is that it is often easy to acquire. However, there are concerns to be considered with self-report data and these concerns should be addressed in the Discussion section. In qualitative and quantitative data, self-report is dependent on a participant's perception, which is not always easily verified or corroborated. Self-report data is subject to several forms of bias, which are limitations that need to be discussed (Brutus, Aguinis, & Wassmer, 2013). Biases may become apparent when DNP students begin to notice incongruences with their data compared with data in published reports. Some of the more typical biases include:

1. **Discerning memory**: Participants may not be able to remember past events, especially if those events are associated with traumatic occurrences.
2. **Telescoping**: Participants may confuse the chronology of an event. For example, recalling events that occurred in the 1960s as if they occurred in the 1970s.
3. **Acknowledgment error**: Participants may attribute positive outcomes to their own behaviors or traits while attributing negative behaviors to an external entity.
4. **Exaggeration**: Participants may inadvertently embellish life events to a greater significance than they really were. Participants may also experience confabulation, a memory disorder in which stories are made up.

Transparency and acknowledgment are essential when self-report issues are noted in DNP project data. Addressing self-report issues will enhance a project's credibility and also inform others on how to possibly avoid self-report issues in similar projects.

Potential Student Limitations

Experienced researchers, academicians, and practitioners are well acquainted with individual experiences that are limitations to studies and projects. It is important to not apologize for these limitations, but instead acknowledge their existence and describe any activities used to compensate for deficits. A few of these limitations include:

Access: At times, and more than likely beyond a student's control, access to participants and settings is limited or denied. Reasons may range from closure of a program to change in staffing patterns. Regardless of the cause, the reason for denied access needs to be described in the project paper.

Time constraints: DNP students generally do not have the time or resources to conduct longitudinal projects. Unforeseeable or uncontrollable events may occur that prohibited a student from adhering to a predetermined timeline. If the timeline is altered and affects the project's outcomes, be certain to document and describe time or resource constraint as a limitation.

Bias: Bias in a DNP project may occur when participants, settings, or events are viewed inaccurately. Bias may take a negative or positive form. It is not uncommon for bias to be present in research studies or DNP projects. Qualitative research has design features included to help limit bias. Be particularly critical when proofreading a DNP paper to evaluate the order and completeness of the project's design. For example, be alert to any possible omissions in data collection or inconsistencies in how participants and settings were portrayed. Any detection of bias needs to be described.

Language: Many DNP projects serve ethnically diverse populations. Be certain to document if the implementation of a project is limited or negatively influenced due to language barriers on the part of the student or project team.

WRITING THE LIMITATIONS SECTION

The limitations description is placed at the beginning of the Discussion section. This placement acknowledges for readers the presence and understanding of limitations prior to reading the interpretations of a project's data analyses. It is important to avoid placing the limitations description in the middle of the Discussion section to prevent the perception of unimportance. As limitations are discussed in the project paper, it is critical to:

- Describe the limitations concisely.
- Explain why the limitations occurred.
- Explain why the limitations could not be avoided.
- Evaluate the influence of the limitations.
- Describe how the limitations could better inform future projects or research.

Remember, a limitations section is not an opportunity to grovel. Instead, identify the limitation and explain how applying a different design approach or methodology might effectively leverage limitations in future projects. See Box 6.4 for key phrases used in writing limitation statements.

BOX 6.4 KEY PHRASES FOR LIMITATION STATEMENTS

- Because of time constraints, it was decided not to explore…
- An additional limitation involves the issue of…
- One concern about the project outcome was…
- The design presented limitations, such as…
- The limitations of this project include…
- Because of the data collection limitations, it could be argued that…

CONCLUSION OF DISCUSSION SECTION

The conclusion is an important capstone that serves as an integrative synopsis to help readers understand why a DNP project matters to patients, healthcare providers, and/or society. The conclusion is not an outline of the paper's main topics but is instead a synthesis of the project's primary points. Usually the conclusion is presented in one well thought-out paragraph. Remember, the introductory statement in the Introduction section provided an opportunity to make a positive first impression. The conclusion provides a final opportunity to create a lasting impression. The conclusion is a means to clearly state the impact that the DNP project had on changing and improving the health of individuals or populations. See Box 6.5 for key phrases used in writing conclusion statements.

BOX 6.5 KEY PHRASES FOR CONCLUSION STATEMENTS

- It is speculated that the primary outcome was related to…
- The primary project outcome seems to depend on…
- The identified problem does seem to improve when…
- This key finding may explain why…

Tables 6.1 and 6.2 prove a review of the discussion section.

Table 6.1

Discussion Section Checklist

Capturing the Discussion in IMRaD

A Discussion section provides the opportunity to describe the importance, significance, applications, and meanings of a DNP project. The discussion section provides fresh insights and understandings about an important clinical or systems topic that was the motivation for beginning the scholarly endeavor.

Discussion I have:	Completed "Yes" or "No"	If "Yes," date completed: If "No," list steps needed to complete:
• Provided a summary of the problem.		
• Reviewed the project's limitations.		
• Emphasized key findings.		
• Described unique characteristics about the sample.		
• Discussed what the project's findings mean in light of what is already know about the problem.		
• Compared and discussed findings in relation to other research and projects.		
• Discussed implications of the findings to practice, education, policy, research, leadership, and/or informatics.		
• Provided sound recommendations for future projects and collaborative research endeavors.		

DNP, Doctor of Nursing Practice; IMRaD, introduction, methodology, results, and discussion.

Table 6.2

Faculty Discussion Table

I have discussed the following Discussion sections with my faculty advisor:	Date discussed	Follow-up.
• References to previous research are logical.	_____	_____
• Explanation of results is sound.	_____	_____
• Limitations are reported.	_____	_____
• Trends and patterns in the data have been adequately identified and described.	_____	_____

SUMMARY

The Discussion section allows for a full elaboration and explanation of a DNP project's results. The Discussion section is a commentary about the project's findings and not a review of analyses and results. The Discussion section provides students an opportunity to describe the project's limitations and recommendations to prevent such limitations in future projects. Importantly, the Discussion section allows students to connect the project findings to clinical implications as well as future projects.

References

Brutus, S., Aguinis, H., & Wassmer, U. (2013). Self-reported limitations and future directions in scholarly reports: Analysis and recommendation. *Journal of Management, 39*(1), 48–75. doi:10.1177/0149206312455245

Joyner, R. L., Rouse, W. A., & Glatthorn, A. A. (2013). *Writing the winning thesis or dissertation: A step-by-step guide*. London, UK: Corwin.

Polit, D. F., & Beck, C. T. (2019). *Essentials of nursing research: Appraising evidence for nursing practice*. Philadelphia, PA: Wolters Kluwer Health/Lippincott Williams & Wilkins.

Roush, K. (2019). *A nurse's step-by-step guide to writing a desertion or scholarly project*. Indianapolis, IN: Sigma Theta Tau International.

7

Completing the DNP Project Paper

After reading this chapter, learners should be able to:

1. Create an effective Doctor of Nursing Practice (DNP) project title.
2. Identify keywords in a DNP project paper.
3. Develop an abstract for a DNP project paper.

INTRODUCTION

A completed Doctor of Nursing Practice (DNP) project paper becomes part of a multifaceted information network. A DNP project's outcomes contribute to the improvement of healthcare and healthcare delivery in a diverse range of settings. In addition to the introduction, methodology, results, and discussion (IMRaD) components, other elements are required to finalize a DNP project paper. The required elements include: (1) title, (2) abstract, (3) table of contents, (4) selecting keywords, (5) acknowledgment and dedication, and (6) appendices. Once a DNP paper is finalized and meets faculty standards for approval of completion, the paper needs to be disseminated in the form of a poster, podium, and/or manuscript.

SELECTING A TITLE

An effective title is a truthful prelude of the project paper's content (Joyner, Rouse, & Glatthorn, 2013). Although the shortest part of a DNP project paper, a title is one of the most critical elements of the project paper. The title is the introduction of a DNP project to readers, reviewers, and editors. Therefore, a title must be selected that garners immediate attention and, with precision, describes the relevant contents of a DNP project paper.

Writing an effective DNP project paper title is challenging and requires time and thought. Writing an effective title requires listing and describing relationships among the major concepts covered in the DNP paper. For example, "low back pain, symptom monitoring, physical activity" may be examples of major concepts, and "Advanced Practice Nurse consultation" may be a mediator that fosters the conceptual relationships or linkages. Each key concept and mediator will need to be included in a title.

It is recommended that titles for scholarly works (e.g., DNP projects, posters, manuscripts) not exceed 12 words. Long titles are frequently awkward and may exasperate readers. It is questionable whether journal editors will accept a manuscript with an excessively long title. When creating a title for a DNP project it is important to consider what will be of interest in a project paper to other nurses and healthcare providers. In addition, students might consider what motivated their interest to conduct a project. Titles that pique a reader's interest and communicate personal motivation are ways to attract and encourage them to read a project paper (Branson, 2004). It may be tempting to use humor and uniqueness in a DNP project title; however, humor and novelty are best used when writing for select audiences.

Consider the following titles:

1. *A Comprehensive Cultural Humility Toolkit for Advanced Practice Nurses Working with Marginalized Populations to Promote a Sense of Acceptance at an Adult Healthcare Clinic in an Urban Neighborhood*

The title is too long, uses irrelevant words, and is clumsy to read. In addition, major concepts and their interrelationships are not easily recognizable.

2. *Cultural Humility: A DNP Project*

The title does not provide all of the key concepts. It offers limited information of interest and does not optimize conceptual linkages.

3. *Positive Effects of Healthcare Provider Cultural Humility Training on Patient Satisfaction for Marginalized Populations*

The title is succinct and presents the relevant concepts and their proposed relationships.

As the title is being developed, students can write several potential options. The options can be shared with faculty, advisors, and peers for critique. Following a critique, a student can select one title and refine it further. Remember, the excellence and content of a project paper will not matter if no one reads the paper. A quality title may compel a potential reviewer to consider reading a manuscript. In addition, a quality title serves to describe upcoming content and establish a scholarly tone for a project paper.

ABSTRACT

An abstract is a summary of a full DNP project paper. An abstract is designed to briefly describe the Introduction, Methodology, Results, and Discussion (IMRaD) sections of the project paper. An effective abstract, although brief, requires careful planning, logical thinking, and concise communication (Pierson, 2004). An abstract succinctly coveys to readers the following information about the project paper:

- Why it was done.
- What was done.
- What was learned.
- Implications of findings.

School faculty will likely have a predetermined standardized length (i.e., number of words) of the abstract. The abstract will mirror the IMRaD format:

Introduction: This is a brief section of the abstract, often two sentences, and answers why the project was undertaken. In this section, the aim of the project will be stated.

Example: The aim of this project was to increase steps walked by persons following coronary artery bypass surgery. Paralytic ileus is a post-surgical complication that may be prevented by early ambulation.

Methods: The Methods section of the abstract answers what was done. In the limited space, often two or three sentences, convey the type of design, setting, sample, and measurements.

Results: In this section, the reader is informed about what was learned from the project. In the limited space provided, convey results using real data. For example, avoid "It was found that X is perceived to be superior to Y." Instead, write "Of the 100 participants, 47% reported a preference for group walking as a form of exercise."

Discussion: This section of the abstract reports implications for practice and future projects. It is a brief statement, one or two sentences, that reports why the project's findings are important. For instance, "The group-walking program can be easily and cost-effectively implemented into various diverse post-surgical environments."

Be sure to use the active voice and simple declarative sentences when writing an abstract. Use generic names for brands and products unless a specific brand was used (Pierson, 2004). Remember, the readers of abstracts will be from widely different disciplines and backgrounds. It may seem safe to use commonplace abbreviations, but it is better not to do so. Simply write out COPD the first time it is used.

TABLE OF CONTENTS

The table of contents is a list of chapters or major sections (e.g., IMRaD) of a DNP project paper.

Fast Facts

A well-formatted and logical table of contents indicates to readers that a quality paper has been prepared.

Place the table of contents after the abstract and before the introduction. Primary elements of a table of contents page include: (1) a page title, (2) headings (e.g., Introduction, Methodology, Results, Discussion) and subheadings, and (3) pagination to indicate where each section of the DNP project paper is located. Include level one and level two headings in the table of contents. Level three headings are omitted if the table of contents exceeds three pages.

Example:

Level one = **Chapter 2 Methodology**
Level two = 2.1 Setting
Level three = 2.1.1 Barriers to Setting

Clear and accurate headings must be used throughout the project paper to enhance a reader's ability to navigate the paper.

SELECTING KEYWORDS

A keyword helps unlock barriers to information. Keywords point readers to pertinent articles they may not usually read. Keywords enable search engines (e.g., MEDLINE, PsycINFO, Cochrane Data Base of Systematic Reviews) to locate relevant articles for students, scholars, and researchers.

Fast Facts

Effective keywords help increase the number of a manuscript's potential readers.

To be effective, keywords must be selected carefully to represent the content of a DNP paper. Keywords must also be specific to the identified problem addressed in the paper. Avoid using words from the paper's title as keywords. When choosing keywords for a DNP paper, select words that:

- Identify specific geographic regions referred to in the DNP paper (e.g., rural healthcare, Southwest border health security).
- Name materials or procedures used in the DNP project (e.g., arthroplasty, insulin, cesarean section).
- Identify settings germane to the project (long-term care facility, hemodialysis unit, hospice).
- Specify phenomena (e.g., food desert, climate change, healthcare literacy).

Consider the following example:

DNP paper title: Positive Effects of Healthcare Provider Cultural Humility Training on Patient Satisfaction for Marginalized Populations

Less effective keywords: Cultural Competence, Advanced Practice Nurses, Isolation

Effective keywords: Belongingness, Patient Engagement, Power Imbalance

Students may want to test their keyword selection. To check keyword selection, enter keywords into a search engine or database to determine if results include publications that are similar to the DNP project.

ACKNOWLEDGMENT AND DEDICATION

Acknowledgments are generally optional. The purpose of an acknowledgment is to thank or acknowledge those who contributed to the DNP project and/or paper in a meaningful way (Polit & Beck, 2019). An acknowledgment appears after the cover page. Do not be overzealous in paying tribute to everyone who made a contribution to a career trajectory. Usually, a student's advisor and members of the advisory group are acknowledged. The acknowledgment needs to match the professional tone of the DNP paper. In the acknowledgment, address each person with their full professional name and title. For example, "I thank my advisor Jane Smith, DNP, RN for her time and guidance throughout the DNP project."

A dedication allows a student to pay tribute to a person or persons who have made special contributions to a student's career and/or project. A dedication is generally not long and needs to be written in the same professional, grammatical style as the paper. Names and titles of people should be written out fully.

APPENDICES

The body of the DNP paper provides a great deal of information to support the DNP project and discuss its salient findings. However, there often will be supplementary information that will not be part of the text but will be useful to share with interested readers. Supplementary information is often detailed and can make the body of the DNP paper excessively long. It is best to move supplementary information to the appendices. The appendices must contain only additional information. Do not include information in an appendix that is critical for understanding the intent and content of the project paper. Content in an appendix may include:

- Additional results: As mentioned in the Results section, analyses, whether quantitative or qualitative, will produce voluminous amounts of data. Data that are less significant to answering the PICOT question or addressing the problem statement may be placed in the appendices.
- Surveys and interview questions: Surveys and interviews do not belong in the main body of a project paper. It is important to include written materials, such as surveys and questionnaires, in an appendix so readers may fully evaluate data collection resources.
- Letters and forms: Letters requesting consent to participate in a project and other institutional review board (IRB) materials need to be placed the appendices. Letters to key stakeholders are also placed in the appendices.
- Tables, figures, charts, and grafts: Tables and illustrations may be too abundant to place in the main body of a project paper. However, they may contain important data and information. These documents belong in the appendices.

It is best to format the appendices into separate components instead of one long appendix. Separating the components (e.g., surveys, letter of consent, field notes) helps to make the information more accessible to readers. Begin each appendix as a new page. Number and title each appendix for clarity in the body of the paper. The appendix section is placed in the paper after the reference list.

DISSEMINATION

The IMRaD format is required for many poster, podium, and publication venues. It is important to determine what the conference or journal expects to be included in each IMRaD section. DNP project papers are quite lengthy and could not possibly be presented in total for any reasonable length of a publication or presentation. It is advisable to work with faculty or experienced authors and/or presenters when preparing to disseminate the findings from a DNP project.

SUMMARY

Writing a DNP project paper requires ambition, patience, and perseverance. A well-organized DNP project paper will include the essential IMRaD sections as well as attention to the other structural elements that contribute to a successful project paper. Students work hard throughout a project process and their papers need to be a reflection of the time and hard work as well as results and, thus, should be presented with integrity befitting a scholarly nurse.

References

Branson, R. D. (2004). Anatomy of a research paper. *Respiratory Care*, *49*(10), 1222–1228.

Joyner, R. L., Rouse, W. A., & Glatthorn, A. A. (2013). *Writing the winning thesis or dissertation: A step-by-step guide*. London, UK: Corwin.

Pierson, D. J. (2004). How to write an abstract that will be accepted for presentation at a national meeting. *Respiratory Care*, *49*(10), 1206–1212.

Polit, D. F., & Beck, C. T. (2019). *Essentials of nursing research: Appraising evidence for nursing practice*. Philadelphia, PA: Wolters Kluwer Health/Lippincott Williams & Wilkins.

Index

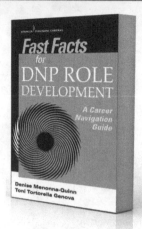
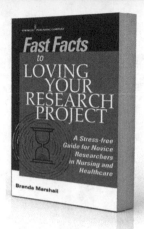
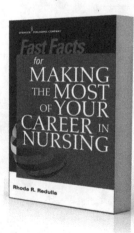
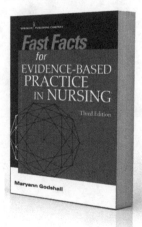